# KARA GOUCHER'S
# RUNNING
# FOR WOMEN

## From First Steps to Marathons

# KARA GOUCHER

### with Adam Bean

**A TOUCHSTONE BOOK**

Published by Simon & Schuster

New York    London    Toronto    Sydney

Touchstone
A Division of Simon & Schuster, Inc.
1230 Avenue of the Americas
New York, NY 10020

First Touchstone trade paperback edition April 2011

TOUCHSTONE and colophon are registered trademarks of Simon & Schuster, Inc.

For information about special discounts for bulk purchases, please contact Simon & Schuster Special Sales at 1-866-506-1949 or business@simonandschuster.com.

The Simon & Schuster Speakers Bureau can bring authors to your live event. For more information or to book an event, contact the Simon & Schuster Speakers Bureau at 1-866-248-3049 or visit our website at www.simonspeakers.com.

Designed by Ruth Lee-Mui

Manufactured in the United States of America

10  9  8  7  6  5  4  3  2

Library of Congress Cataloging-in-Publication Data

Goucher, Kara.
 Kara Goucher's running for women : from first steps to marathons / by Kara Goucher with Adam Bean.
  p. cm.
 "A Touchstone Book."
 Includes index.
 1. Running for women. 2. Marathon running—Training. I. Bean, Adam. II. Title.
GV1061.18.W66G68  2010
796.42082—dc22          2010050144

ISBN 978-1-4391-9612-0
ISBN 978-1-4391-9613-7 (ebook)

This book is dedicated to everyone who has played a part in my journey through running. From former teammates and assistant coaches to fellow road racers and competitors. A special dedication to my husband Adam, my mother Patty Wheeler, my grandparents Cal and Ola Jean Haworth, my sisters Kelly Wheeler and Kendall Schoolmeester, and to all of my coaches, who have cultivated my love for the sport: Coach Dick Skogg, Mark Wetmore, and Alberto Salazar.

# ACKNOWLEDGMENTS

We would like to thank the following runners and experts for their gracious, invaluable help with this book:

Robin Barrett, MD

Madeleine Bean

Sophie Bean

Dan Bernadot, PhD

Ruth Carey, RD

Kristine Clark, PhD

Nancy Clark, MS, RD

Jim Denison, PhD

Editors of *Runner's World* magazine

Editors of *Runner's World–UK* magazine

Matt Fitzgerald

Susan Kleiner, PhD

Al Kupczak

Allison Lind, DPT

Megan McMorris

Joe Mills, PhD

Stephen Pribut, DPM

Alberto Salazar

Tony Salazar

Darren Treasure, PhD

Justin Whittaker, DC

Mark Will-Weber

# CONTENTS

# INTRODUCTION

What I hope to do in this book is the same thing my early running mentors did for me: help you gain a lifelong passion for running. I am not a coach. I have no fancy scientific training methodologies to offer. But I do think I'm a good role model for other women runners and *potential* women runners. In what way? I have mastered the art of being in love with running. Always have been. Always will be.

In these pages I hope to mentor you in this art by way of personal stories and advice. At the beginning of each chapter, I briefly describe a particular aspect of my life in running. I talk about what has worked for me and what hasn't, my setbacks (I've had lots) and my accomplishments. I share experiences I've had with training, racing, building a support network, and dealing with difficult episodes of emotional eating. Finally, I share my hopes for the future, which go way beyond my current status as a professional distance runner. I hope you find these life dispatches inspiring and informative.

Each chapter then segues into what this book is really all about, which is running advice aimed directly at you, to help you become a better, happier, healthier, more fulfilled runner. I know how busy you are. If you're like me, you rarely have much time for actual reading anymore, which is why I wanted to make it easy for you to get something substantive from this book every time you pick it up—even if it's just for a minute or two. Thus the reliance on short, quickly "digested" tips, strategies, and pearls of running wisdom. Hundreds of them, in fact. Each one is another potential reason to fall in love with running as I have done.

Best of luck. I hope I'll see you on the roads.

KARA GOUCHER'S
# RUNNING
# FOR WOMEN

# CHAPTER 1

# GETTING STARTED

love to run. I am crazy, madly, head-over-heels in love with running.

My love affair started when I was a little girl growing up in Minnesota in a house full of women, always competing for bathroom time with my older sister, Kelly, born two years before me; my younger sister, Kendall, who came along four years after me; and our strong, compassionate, competitive mom. We moved to Duluth from New York City when I was four, not long after my father was killed on the road by a drunk driver. My mom's parents lived there and she wanted their help in raising my sisters and me, which they were glad to offer.

Papa, as we called our mom's dad, was a runner. When I was six, he took me to a local 1-mile fun run. I remember standing at the starting line with Papa and hearing the starting horn sound. I guess I was too slow to react because I was immediately run over from behind. I got up with a bloody knee. Papa expected me to freak out.

"Let's go get that cleaned up," he said.

I did freak out, but not for the reason Papa thought I would.

"We're getting left behind!" I shouted, pointing at the other runners scampering away from us. "Let's go! Let's go!"

So we ran. Only after we finished did I get a Band-Aid for my knee. Papa was proud of me. He wanted his granddaughters to become strong women like his wife and daughter. He didn't see any reason why resilience shouldn't be encouraged in girls as it was in boys.

For a long time after that first race, running was just one of many activities I enjoyed. Mom believed in giving my sisters and me a variety of experiences, and I went with the flow. I took lessons in dancing, French horn, painting, sculpture, and more, and I played soccer, baseball, tennis, and softball, among other sports. I practically lived in the family minivan going from one activity to another.

In the fourth grade I ran another 1-mile kids' run that was connected to a big Mother's Day 5K race in Duluth, which still exists. I was the first girl to finish, and only four boys beat me. The next year I ran it again and lost to another girl. That really irritated me. I brooded for days.

It was pretty obvious that I had inherited my mother's competitiveness. She has a steely will to win that is usually hidden behind a big, soft heart that she wears on her sleeve. Because Mom isn't an athlete or a high-powered business executive, it comes out in funny ways. When Mom and my sisters and I made Christmas cookies together, she took pride in making the best-decorated cookies, and she insisted that they be placed at the bottom of the Tupperware container, to be eaten last.

Sharing my mom's distaste for losing, I was determined to avenge my loss in the Mother's Day 5K kids' fun run, and the following May I did. Sort of. I was now too old to do the kids' run, so I ran the full 5K and won my age group. By this time, running had begun to separate itself from the many other hobbies in my life. It gave me a special satisfaction, maybe because it came to me more naturally than anything else I had ever tried. So in the seventh grade I joined my junior high cross-country team. I improved with every race and won the city championship. My performance there made an impression on our high school track coach, Mr. Skogg, who invited me to try out for the track team in the spring, two years early (which is allowed in my home state).

I've been a runner ever since, and Coach Skogg is one big reason. He was not what you might expect a great high school track coach to be. He had never been a runner and was built like a shot-putter. An aroma of coffee and cigars followed him everywhere. He did not know much about exercise physiology, and most of what he knew about training for distance running came from his *Runner's World* subscription. Coach Skogg never talked about times and paces. In fact, he did not seem to really care how fast we ran or if we improved. I ran all my best times as a ninth grader and never got any faster in my last three

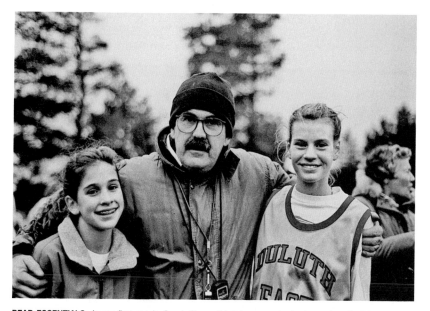

**BEAR ESSENTIALS:** As my first coach, Coach Skogg didn't know much about exercise physiology and got most of his training information from *Runner's World* magazine, but he was well known—and much beloved—for the bear hugs he gave all his runners at the finish line. Here I am with Coach Skogg and my teammate Amy Hill, now Amy Oldenberg.

years of high school, which bothered me a little, but it did not bother Coach Skogg.

What made him a great coach was not the results he produced in his runners; it was the fun we had running for him. I used to look forward to practice all day at school. Coach created a relaxed environment that was all about camaraderie, laughter, and the joy of running. He was like another grandfather to most of us. At the end of each race, he would give us bear hugs as we came through the finish chute one by one. It didn't matter how well or poorly we had run—we always got the same hug.

When I graduated from Duluth East High School in 1996, I couldn't have imagined all the experiences running would bring me in the coming years: among them, winning college national championships, signing a professional contract with Nike, being coached by the legendary Alberto Salazar, winning a World Championship medal, qualifying for and competing in two events in one Olympics, and not least of all, finding the other great love of my life, my husband, Adam, who happens to be one of the best American runners of our generation.

It hasn't all been smooth sailing. There have been many times when I have struggled in my running. I have dealt with injuries. I have wilted under the pressure to perform. And more than once I have let my competitiveness get out of hand. But through it all, my love of running has never left me. At the very least, running has always been a relief and a sanctuary—something that makes me feel good, both physically and mentally. This pure enjoyment is really more important to me than winning races and even more important than the great blessing of being able to make a living as a runner. I would love running just as much if I had never won anything, and I will continue to enjoy running long after I can no longer make a living at it.

I am not sure I would love running if I had not gotten started the way I had, though. I was very lucky to have mentors who taught me that running was supposed to be fun and fulfilling. Papa showed me how running can create a bond with other people and how satisfying it is to push your body and see what it can do, whether you're fast or slow. Coach Skogg showed me that running can be the highlight of your day, every day, and that running for pure pleasure is the surest way to run well.

When you love something as much as I love running, it is natural to want to share it. The older I get, the more strongly I feel the desire to help other people—especially other women—fall in love with running. For me it's not so much about the health benefits. Those are great, but I believe that the best thing about running is the joy it brings to life. In any case, only if you love running will you keep doing it long enough to maximize those health benefits. If you put your enjoyment of running first, the rest takes care of itself, whether you're trying to lose weight, strengthen your bones, or win an Olympic gold medal. I really believe that.

Ready to get started? Great. I'm here to help.

# SIMPLE TIPS FOR GETTING YOU OFF ON THE RIGHT FOOT

No matter your age, your exercise background, or your current fitness level, you can become a runner. Before the fitness revolution of the 1970s and 1980s, pretty much everyone who ran was young and fast. That's not the case anymore. Today you see all shapes and sizes out on the roads, and no one thinks a thing of it.

Some people are in it to get fast (I guess I'm one of them!), but these days people run for all sorts of reasons—all of them *good* reasons. You want to feel better? You want more energy? You need to lose a few pounds? Reduce your stress level? Running helps with all those things and so much more.

One of the best things is that you don't need much to get started, apart from desire. And a little bit of guidance. The following tips and strategies should do the trick.

**GET THE OKAY FROM YOUR DOCTOR:** Just to be on the safe side, it's important to get a checkup before starting a running program. You don't want to be surprised by a condition that might be dangerous or that could hamper your running effort.

**ENTER WITH NO WORRIES WHATSOEVER:** Some sports and activities take pride in their "apartness." They're like clubs—with passwords and secret handshakes—and only the select few are allowed inside. Running is not like that. *Runners* are not like that. We tend to be an open-minded, whatever-you're-in-it-for-is-fine-with-me group. It's all about what motivates you, whether that's competition, health, weight control, meeting guys at races, or darn near anything else. Running is open to people of all shapes, sizes, ages, and abilities.

## I LOVE THIS QUOTE

Have a dream, make a plan, go for it. You'll get there, I promise.
—Zoe Koplowitz, Achilles Track Club member with
multiple sclerosis who required 24 hours on crutches
but finished the 1993 New York City Marathon

I love this quote because I do believe that anything is possible. Dream big, have faith, and believe.

**DON'T BE SCARED:** Okay, admittedly, running can be a little intimidating, especially if you have never been an athlete and are worried if you have what it takes. Well, I'm here to say you do. I once had as many doubts about running as you did, until I realized I was just as capable as anyone else. That's how I want you to feel.

**AIM FOR 150:** For optimal health, the federal government recommends 30 minutes of aerobic exercise five or more times a week—for example,

7

a 3-mile run at a 10-minute-per-mile pace five days a week. A great goal to shoot for! (But take your time working up to it.)

**MAKE RUNNING A PRIORITY AND YOU'LL FIND THE TIME:** I know plenty of people who are living proof that you can find time to run even with a job and a family. One of them is my brother-in-law Bret. He has a wife, a daughter, and a demanding job that requires him to travel a lot. But he finds time to run. Sure, he has to get creative to squeeze in workouts—for example, by running to work sometimes. But he is willing to do what it takes to keep running because he loves it, so it's a priority for him. That's the key. You'll always find time for something you love.

**LET THE IMPORTANT PEOPLE IN YOUR LIFE KNOW YOUR PLAN TO BECOME A RUNNER:** Some people like to start running on the sly, real low-key like. And that's fine—no need to make a major trumpets-blaring production out of it. But "going public" with your intentions is going to help you stick with it. It keeps you "on the hook." Call it creating positive peer pressure.

**WRITE DOWN YOUR GOAL, BUT DON'T HESITATE TO REVISE IT:** Similarly to letting others know of your plan to start running, it's important to write your running goal(s) down. This may seem silly, but it's not. Writing it down is a signal that you mean business, that it's not a passing fancy.

**RUN FOR TIME, NOT SPEED OR DISTANCE:** Those latter two have their place, but maybe not yet. In the beginning, it's simplest to just get out there for a set period of time. And don't even worry about running the whole time—just be out there. "I'm just going out for 20 minutes" is the way you might think about it. As you become fitter (see page 36 to help you do this), you'll be able to do more and more running when you're out there, and less and less walking.

**TALK YOUR WAY THROUGH IT:** New runners sometimes make the mistake of thinking it's not "real" running unless it's painful and you're gasping for breath. Not true. Use the talk test—the ability to hold a normal conversation with yourself!—to let you know if you're running easily enough. If you can't talk, slow down.

**REMEMBER, YOU ARE A RUNNER NO MATTER WHAT ANYONE SAYS:** Or a person who runs—take your pick! Point being, there's no litmus test for being a runner and no arbiter. You are a runner when you say (and believe) you are a runner. Period.

# I LOVE THIS QUOTE

God has given me the ability. The rest is up to me. Believe.
Believe. Believe . . .
> —Billy Mills, an entry in his training diary prior to his upset
> Olympic gold medal 10,000-meter win in the Tokyo Olympics

I love this quote because I love that Billy put faith in himself. This is what I strive to be like as an athlete.

**RUN SLOWER THAN YOU EVER HAVE IN YOUR LIFE:** Some women are intimidated by running because they think they'll start breathing too hard, in part because they remember that's how running was back in gym class. Unfortunately, old-fashioned gym teachers—many of whom used running as a punishment for bad behavior—turned a lot of people off to running. But you're not in gym anymore and things have changed. You control when, where, and how fast you run. So if you start breathing hard, just slow down or take a walk break.

**KEEP YOUR TOENAILS TRIMMED:** Okay, maybe a little gross, but toes can take a beating when you run. If your toenails are too long, they'll jam up against your running shoes with each step. Not good.

9

**BUY NICE SOCKS:** Running socks sometimes get lost in all the hype surrounding running shoes. Socks are important, too! They're next to your skin; your shoes aren't. Make sure they're *running* socks, not tennis or soccer socks, because running socks are normally synthetic (one exception is SmartWool socks—very comfy) for better moisture management. Consider those with extra padding on the bottom. Or, if you're prone to blisters, try thinner socks. They'll cause less friction inside your shoes.

**WEAR SYNTHETIC SPORT OR RUNNING SOCKS:** This will ensure proper fit, moisture wicking, and support. Casual cotton socks won't cut it, especially on wet days, when cotton or wool will definitely increase your blister risk.

**RUN FOR FUN, OR TO RACE:** Some people see running as a sport, with competition as its raison d'être. Others see running as an activity, with things like health, stress relief, and weight control as the point of the activity. Actually, running is all those things—and many more besides. Take your pick.

**OVERCOME SELF-CONSCIOUSNESS:** One thing that stops a lot of people from becoming runners—or staying in the sport—is that they don't want to be seen running in their own neighborhood! They think they look slow, or fat, or old, or sweaty, or whatever. Don't let any of that stop you! Among runners, you are golden. Running deserves respect, and every runner knows it and shows it toward his or her fellow runner.

**WEAR A RUNNING SKIRT:** You've probably seen runners wearing these. They're very flattering. They've been around about five years and are getting more and more popular. The underpants part of the skirt cinches you in a bit, and the skirt part is kind of wrap-like and doesn't cling like shorts can. They're comfortable, too. Another option is tights, which cover your legs a bit if you're self-conscious at all. You can get half tights, too, which come down to your knees and are a bit cooler than full-length tights.

**ICE WITH A FROZEN GEL PACK OR A BAG OF FROZEN PEAS:** As a runner, you will occasionally experience a little pain and swelling, perhaps from a twisted ankle or sore shins. It comes with the territory. Icing for 15 to 20 minutes (no more) can help a lot, but forget the ice cubes in a towel routine. Gel packs that you keep in the freezer conform better, and they usually come with strips or a "sleeve" for better compression against the sore area. You can get them at any sports or running store. Or the next time you're at the grocery store, get a bag of frozen corn or peas. Perfect for icing sore body parts—and reusable, of course.

**GET RID OF THAT STITCH:** A side stitch is a cramp, usually on your right side. Stitches are common among new runners but rare among veteran runners. Several possible causes include muscle spasming, lack of oxygen to the GI muscles, internal organs pulling down on the diaphragm muscle, and so on. More to the point, it hurts and it's hard to run through it. Two methods for combating stitches are (1) exhale forcefully while bending over at the waist (admittedly not pretty) and (2) press your fingers into the painful area. A third method probably works best of all: stop and walk until the stitch goes away. Many new runners find if they avoid eating any solid food just before a run, they get stitches less frequently.

**SHOO AWAY SHIN SPLINTS:** Shin splits are more common for beginners than stitches and unfortunately they take longer to get rid of. You'll sometimes feel shin splint pain in the inside or the outside edge of the shin. That's because shin splints are caused by the muscles on the front of the leg essentially pulling away from the shin, resulting in pain and inflammation. Sometimes tight calves are a contributing cause, but it's normally just a case of the shin muscles not being used to the stress of running; thus shin splints are a little like growing pains in children. The good news is that they normally respond quickly to rest and twice-a-day icing. Don't try to run through them, though, as they can really hang on unless you deal with them. A good home exercise for preventing and recovering from shin splints is to sit in a chair and write out the entire alphabet on the floor with your pointed foot. Switch legs and do the same with the other foot. This simple exercise does wonders for the muscles around your shins. Recovering from a bad bout of shin splints? Do the letters in capitals first, then again in lowercase!

**DON'T OVERTHINK IT:** As with any other activity, there's plenty of running minutiae to obsess about if that's your thing. And the terms can be awfully impressive: lactate threshold training, overpronation, running economy, interval training, tempo running, and one of my personal favorites—VO2 max. But in the end, you'll do just fine as a runner with a few basic training principles. There's a lot to be said for keeping things simple.

**TRY TO HAVE A SIMPLE GAME PLAN FOR EVERY RUN:** Nothing elaborate here, but it's really good to know what you plan to accomplish before you head out the door. A simple statement of intent works best, and you might even say it out loud.

- "I just need to get out for some fresh air for 30 minutes."
- "I want to fit in 8 to 10 pickups to work on my speed a little."
- "I will do 4 miles *easy.* That's it."
- "I just need to stretch out my legs after my race yesterday."
- "I want to burn some extra calories after last night's pig-out session."

**CHANGE YOUR RUNNING GOAL IF THE PURSUIT OF IT BECOMES STRESSFUL:** There's positive stress and there's negative stress. Positive stress is the occasional anxiety and excitement you might feel in training for your first 5K race or your first marathon. As long as you don't become a basketcase, this goal is fine. You'll feel all that much better about accomplishing it knowing it wasn't always easy along the way. But running your first 5K or marathon could end up being the wrong goal at the wrong time if it causes too much stress. No one but you will be able to make this call. So try to be open to the possibility that it could go either way, and know that either way will be the right way.

# I LOVE THIS QUOTE

Mental will is a muscle that needs exercise, just like the muscles of the body.

—Lynn Jennings, three-time World Cross Country Champion

I love this quote because Lynn hits the nail on the head. You have to work on your mental toughness. It is just like everything else you do in training; you must work on it to perfect it.

**DON'T WORRY ABOUT FOOD AND DRINK:** Sure, there are lots of ways that smart eating and drinking can enhance your running, and we'll get into all that in Chapter 6. But really, for beginners at least, running nutrition is pretty much the same as walking nutrition. And you don't obsess about what to eat or drink before going out for a walk, do you?

**BYPASS THE MARATHON IF YOU WANT:** Something strange has occurred with the marathon. It has recently become much more accessible thanks to open-to-all beginner marathon training programs, walk/run marathon programs, walker-friendly marathon races that have no finishing time limits, and so on. This is all fine, but what's happened in some social circles is the marathon has become *so* accessible that, you know, you're a loser if you haven't done one. Totally not true. The marathon isn't

13

GETTING STARTED

for everyone, so don't feel like you have to do one to prove your worth as a runner.

## DEAR KARA

**Do you think it's okay to wear only a jog bra on hot days or do I need a top over it?**

I think it's great to wear a sports bra without a top on hot days. It shows that you have a good healthy body image. I must warn you, however: I have worn a sports bra only for years. I have a permanent sports bra tan line!

**HEAD OUT IN THE RAIN:** These can be the best runs of all. Just wear a brimmed hat to keep the rain out of your eyes and tight-fitting synthetic clothing that won't hang on you and get heavy.

**DRESS LIKE IT'S 10 DEGREES WARMER THAN THE THERMOMETER SAYS:** You may feel a little cold at first, but a mile into your run you'll be glad you dressed lightly.

**KEEP IT LAYERED IN COLD WEATHER:** You'll soon learn you don't need to wear much to stay warm on a run, except on the bitterest days (20 degrees and below). It's best to have a thin synthetic wicking layer next to your skin, then—if the temperature is below 50 or so—a tight-weave shell-like layer on top. On wet days, this outer layer should be water resistant if not waterproof. Otherwise, a long-sleeve running T-shirt will be adequate, along with the under layer. On cold days, you'll probably need tights or noncotton sweats on the bottom and perhaps a third middle layer on top for insulation. Use hats, headbands, gloves, or mittens as needed to protect your extremities.

**HAVE A BACKUP FOR REALLY CRAPPY WEATHER:** If you just can't face it outside, have an indoor option to fall back on. The treadmill in the basement; a quick trip to the gym; running in place, alternating with jumping rope, alternating with home stair-climbing (that's right, *real* stair-climbing!). Just keep moving for a minimum of 15 to 20 minutes and you'll feel a lot better, and you won't have missed a day.

**FIND A LOCAL HIGH SCHOOL TRACK AND MAKE IT YOUR FALL-BACK FRIEND:** In terms of always knowing what you're getting and having a controlled running environment, a track is like a treadmill—but better. Better because it's not *quite* so controlled, plus you're outside. A track is perfect for beginners for several reasons:

- The surface is even and generally softer than cement.
- You usually have other runners to keep you company.
- It's easy to keep track of your distance.
- It's fun to throw in half-lap pickups or sprints on the straightaways.
- You can really zone out without getting lost.

**BETTER YET, TRY TO RUN ON THREE SURFACES EACH WEEK—ROAD, TRAIL, AND TRACK:** The first is easy: the streets in your neighborhood. The second you'll find in most nearby parks, or if you're lucky you have state or national parks close by. And the third is found at most high schools. Running on these three surfaces ensures your running scenery will vary, and your feet and legs will get a better workout on the different terrain.

**SUBSCRIBE TO A RUNNING MAGAZINE:** The best of the best is *Runner's World*, which has been informing and inspiring runners of all abilities since 1966. What—you thought it was only for fast runners? Absolutely not, despite what those beautiful people on the cover might imply.

**TRY TO RECOGNIZE WHEN A ROUTINE BECOMES A RUT:** Getting in a same old, same old rut is certainly not just a beginner thing, but it's more com-

15

GETTING STARTED

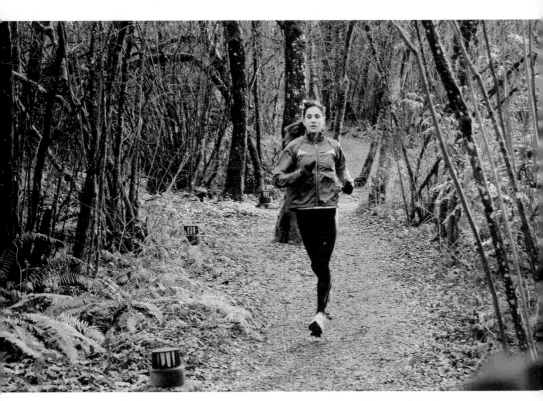

**TRAIL WAYS:** I do frequent off-road running to give my legs a break and get some fresh air.

mon because newbie runners tend to find things that work and hold on tight. That's fine and totally understandable, but at any stage of your running career, keep this in mind: A routine is enjoyable; a rut is not. So you want to be doing the former. A routine is a framework that evolves over time, but at any given point, it is serving its purpose in a positive, functional manner. A rut doesn't evolve, and as opposed to being a framework, it's more like a prison. If you're feeling trapped these days, switch things up. Here are a few suggestions:

- Change the time of day of one of your runs each week.
- Take a short drive or bike ride to a nearby park and run there.
- Do your normal training run, but run it in the opposite direction.
- Add some light speedwork each week in the middle of a regular run.

- Visit the local running shop and see when they do group runs from the store—then go.
- Buy a new running outfit and promise to take on a different run every time you wear it.

**GO EASY MOST OF THE TIME:** There are two main categories of runs: hard runs and easy runs. Hard runs are things like tempo running (I'll explain later in this chapter), hills, interval running on the track (ditto, more on this later), that sort of thing. Easy runs are . . . easy runs! Happily, even if you start training for races and get serious about competition, they're also the type of runs you need to do most often. As long as you keep the pace comfortable and avoid running farther than you are ready to go, these runs will give your body a solid foundation. Actually, as a new runner, all your runs should be easy runs until you have created your foundation, then you can move on to more challenging runs. Or not. Some runners only do easy running for their entire lives, and that's fine, too!

**GO EASY MOST OF THE TIME, PART II:** Even advanced runners do more easy runs than any other type of run. For example, in a typical week, I run thirteen times, and nine of those runs are easy. But when you reach a certain level, easy runs don't really build fitness anymore; they maintain the fitness you've already built. At this point, it's your harder runs that will take your fitness higher. Easy runs should be fun. For me, they are a chance to chat with running partners or listen to music and zone out. Training would not be nearly as fun if I didn't have these runs to balance out my tough workouts.

**INCLUDE LONG RUNS OCCASIONALLY:** I'll mention long runs several times in this book because they're so important. Once you get to the level where your body can handle them, long runs will do wonders for your endurance. Of course, "long" means different things to different run-

17

ners. As a general rule, your long runs should account for about 20 percent of your weekly mileage. So if you build up to running 15 miles a week, your long run would be about 3 miles. If you run 30 miles a week, it would be 6 miles. As for pace, it should be about the same as your easy runs, if not slightly slower. I typically do one long run a week, but many runners do them only once every two or three weeks.

**REWARD YOURSELF AT THE END OF EACH WEEK:** Whatever resonates for you as an incentive, do it. A second glass of wine? Sleeping in an extra hour on Saturday morning? A Friday night bath? A massage from your spouse? Whatever it is, have it lined up by Wednesday so that you know what's coming.

**SET THE RIGHT TEMPO:** Many exercise physiologists believe that so-called tempo runs are the best way to improve your running. Tempo runs are sustained runs at a challenging but controlled pace, which in essence is about midway between your easy jogging pace and your sprinting pace. Sometimes tempo pace is described as "comfortably hard," which I think is a great way to think of it. Their purpose is to train your body to run relatively fast for long periods of time. It's important to remember that you should not finish a tempo run feeling exhausted. If this happens, you've either gone too fast or too far. After a tempo workout, you should feel like you could've done more. I include tempo running in some of the training schedules in Chapter 7.

**HAVE FUN (AND GET FIT) LIKE THE SWEDES DO:** There's a great running term that never fails to get a chuckle from new runners: *fartlek*. It's actually a Swedish word for "speedplay," and it's a very effective way to train for runners of all abilities, including beginners. In its most basic form, it's about changing speeds during a run, but never to the point of exhaustion. Rather, it's almost like what little kids do on a playground where they're constantly moving—jogging and fast walking mostly, but with occasional free-spirited sprinting. Thus, "speedplay."

**HEED THE SWEDES, PART II:** To be a little more specific about *fartlek*, the idea is to throw short bursts of speed into an otherwise easy run. You can pick it up for either a designated period of time—30 seconds, 1 minute, whatever—or pick landmarks to race toward. It's a great way to add variety and a wonderful, child-like sense of speed to your running. All the while, you'll be boosting your fitness more than if you simply did steady-state easy running. What's not to love?

**GO WATCH A LOCAL ROAD RACE:** I guarantee this will get you psyched about running. Seriously, it can be so moving. Near the finish is the best viewing spot for witnessing pure emotion, but midrace can be excellent, too, as well as the top of big hills. Remember to cheer like crazy. And remember to bring some Kleenex.

**SPEND THE MONEY ON A GOOD SPORTS BRA (OR TWO OR THREE):** After your running shoes, a sports bra is probably your most important piece of running equipment. And just like your running shoes, if your sports bra fits right, you won't notice it. It's only when it fits poorly that you notice. Here are five buying tips to ensure you get the right sports bra for your body type:

1. **Try on at least three.** Before you head to the dressing room, grab three sizes to try on—the cup size you normally wear, one that's smaller, and one that's larger. Different brands come in slightly different sizes.
2. **Check the straps.** They shouldn't dig into the skin or move around. Rather, somewhere in the middle.
3. **Check the base.** The bra's base band should feel snug (but not too snug) and lie flat all the way around your torso. If the band rides up in the back, you may need to adjust the straps or get a larger size.

4. **Take an overall view.** Have a look at the front, back, and sides. If there's any bunching or wrinkling of the material, you may need a smaller size. If skin is bulging out anywhere, try one size larger.

5. **Jog in place.** Do this for 10 seconds to see if you feel supported. Check to see that the bra stays in place.

## ON THE CONTRARY

**Don't feel like you have to be forced to use only running gear.** I've personally never been a huge fan of the running short and find yoga-type shorts much more comfortable.

**A lot of people like to wear their running shoes all of the time, but this actually breaks them down faster.** I never wear the current pair I'm training in for just walking around.

**MEET THE PENGUIN:** If you've never read any of John "The Penguin" Bingham's columns or heard him give a prerace talk, check him out at JohnBingham.com. Once an overweight smoker and heavy drinker, Bingham started running when he was forty-three and it completely transformed his life. He's been writing about it ever since. He's a funny, insightful, motivating spokesperson for all runners, but especially for those not gifted with great speed. Or any speed. His most famous running aphorism: "The miracle isn't that I finished. The miracle is that I had the courage to start."

**FAST FORWARD YOUR FITNESS WITH INTERVALS:** Training runs called intervals have been around for decades, and you might even consider them shortcuts to getting faster. But it's a pretty intense ride along the way! That said, don't shy away from them (at least eventually, when you're ready for them), because (1) the pain doesn't last long; (2) they're great to do with training partners, because everyone—ahem—suffers together; (3) you'll feel exhilarated afterward; and (4) they'll get you in shape (physically and mentally) better and faster than any other training method. They consist of a series of relatively short, fast intervals or repeats, with brief rest periods between them for recovery. They're traditionally done on a track, but you can do them anywhere that there's a flat, even, measured surface (well-groomed trails are perfect). If you're a beginner, it's best to get used to running and build up your endurance for at least two to three months before adding intervals to your program.

**HEAD FOR THE HILLS:** Hill running makes you strong—period. Hills give you the strength to hold your form together when you're tired, like at the end of a tough run or a race. For example, it's one thing to be fast, but it's another thing to be fast in the last 100 yards of a marathon. I know this all too well! In the 2009 Boston Marathon, I rounded the last corner tied for first place with two other women. I finished third.

**...AND CONSIDER THIS WHEN YOU GET THERE:** Hill training can simply be done over hilly terrain so that you get the benefit "organically," or you can do hills more like interval workouts, with more repetitive structure. With the latter, you warm up, run hard uphill for a certain distance, jog slowly back down the hill to recover, and repeat as many times as the workout calls for. Then you do an easy jog for a cooldown. You can do shorter, steeper hills, which emphasize muscular strength, or longer, more gradual hills, which do wonders for your endurance. I like to do a "ladder" session that includes both types. It goes like this: 200 meters, 300m, 400m, 600m, 400m, 300m, 200m, and I jog back down to the start after each of those repeats. That's a butt-kicker!

**CHECK OUT THE TREADMILL:** Some runners think running on the treadmill isn't real running. I disagree. I don't happen to like treadmill run-

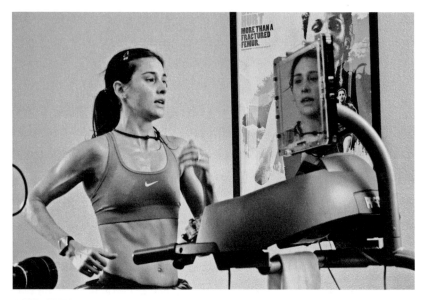

**INSIDE ADDITION:** I use treadmill running as an excellent option on bad-weather days, and when I'm looking for a tightly controlled workout.

ning very much (understatement of the year), but it is most definitely running. And there are several ways you can make it more fun, including:

- **Change speeds.** This may be the best of all. In my experience, what really makes treadmill time slow down is when you do steady-state running. You feel like 5 minutes have passed and look at your watch, and it's been 90 seconds. So mix it up with 2 minutes easy, 2 minutes fast, until you've completed 10 minutes. Same thing with changing the incline. It mixes things up and the time passes more quickly.
- **Run with a buddy on the machine next to you.** This way you can kill time in conversation. Alternatively, take turns changing speed or incline, whereby the other person has to match it. A classic follow-the-leader workout.
- **Watch TV.** A no-brainer—literally—but if it passes the time, so be it.
- **Listen to music.** The treadmill may well be the best place of all to listen to music, as it's safe, the surface is even, there's no traffic to worry about, and it helps with boredom.

**STAY ON THE LEFT:** If you have to run on the road (trails and paths are better and safer), stay as far over on the shoulder as possible, and run facing traffic so that you can see what's coming at you.

**MAKE YOURSELF VISIBLE:** Most running shoes and a lot of running clothing come with reflectivity, but that's not enough. A vest is probably best, as it offers reflectivity on a large surface area. You can easily find one that fits well and looks nice, and that you can put on quickly (no tying or snapping). If you plan to do a lot of night running, especially on roads, also buy a small flashing light that clips on your shorts or that is already attached to a running hat (running stores carry these).

# DEAR KARA

**There's a great city park trail near my house that I love to run on, especially in the early morning. My husband thinks I should never run there alone. I think it's fine. Who is right?**

This is a good question. I used to go to a nature park near my house that has miles and miles of single-track trails. I would go alone and wear my headphones. This bothered my husband to no end. He would be so worried that someone would hurt me or that I would hurt myself and not be able to get help. I think there is a good balance of doing what you love but also being smart. I no longer run on that trail alone. I love running there, but my husband made a lot of good points, and now I only run there when I'm with someone else. If the park you are running in is fairly busy and you see other runners while you are out and about, I don't see any reason to not continue with your routine. But if it is early dusk and you are all alone, you might want to start recruiting a running buddy. It's always better to be safe than sorry.

23

**GO FOR 10 MINUTES IF THAT'S ALL YOU HAVE!** Running is not an all-or-nothing commitment each day. If you have 30 minutes of running on the schedule but can't fit it in or feel too tired to do it, run for 10 minutes instead. Too many women (men, too, of course) think if they can't do their intended workout, then they won't do anything at all. Doesn't have to be like that.

**BEWARE OF UNEVEN STRESSES ON YOUR LEGS:** If you vary the places and surfaces where you run, you'll be fine, but sometimes new runners frequent the same road or the same track every time they run, which can cause problems. For example, if you always run on the left side of the road but your favorite road happens to be highly cambered (on a slant), then your left foot will drop slightly lower than your right with each step. This can eventually lead to pain or even injury. Same goes for running on a track if you're always going in the same direction. The answer is to mix up where you run so that you spread the physical stresses around evenly.

**CONSIDER KEEPING A TRAINING LOG:** You can get these in booklet form or keep your training data online. Logs are useful tools for keeping track of your progress—or lack thereof. It's happened countless times that runners can't figure out what went wrong in a race, or how they got injured, until they review their logs and the secret is revealed.

**KEEP IT FUN:** I used to get bored with my runs when I was growing up in Duluth, Minnesota. My family lived in a neighborhood with a 1-mile running loop right out the front door. I ran that loop over and over until I never wanted to see it again. Like a lot of new runners, I was not comfortable exploring new routes, so I just put up with it until I got smarter and found ways to mix it up. First I did the loop in the opposite direction (obvious, I know!). Then I started playing with my pace, inserting 1-minute speed bursts into some runs and fast finishes into others. Actually, I still use these boredom-busting methods today.

**WAVE TO RUNNERS THAT YOU PASS:** This is an old custom among us. Let's keep it going.

**WAVE TO ONCOMING CARS AS WELL—OR GIVE A HALE AND HEARTY THUMBS-UP:** In a way, this is more important than waving to fellow runners for two important reasons:

1. **It acknowledges that you know you are sharing the road.** Some drivers don't like to share the road. Or they're just worried that they're so close to you, and it freaks them out. Basically your wave or thumbs-up is a way of saying, "Hey, thanks for being okay with me being here."
2. **It gets the driver's attention.** Always a good thing, especially if he or she has been driving along like a space cadet and doesn't register "runner on shoulder" until you break into their consciousness. This happens a lot. You can tell because you think they've seen you, yet when they get close they lurch the wheel to the left as if you had suddenly beamed down from the *Starship Enterprise*.

**STAY CALM IF SOMEONE YELLS AT YOU FROM A PASSING CAR:** Or worse, throws something at you. Granted, it's dangerous and very, very annoying, but you are in no position to challenge this kind of idiotic behavior. Get

## DEAR KARA

**I'm pretty slow and this embarrasses me when I'm running in my neighborhood. Should I run somewhere else (my preference) or just learn to deal with it?**
You need to do what makes you comfortable. You should not feel embarrassed about running slowly; you should be proud that you are out there running! But if that embarrassment is taking the joy out of running, then go somewhere else. Running is a gift in your life and you should enjoy it. If that means going to run somewhere else, then so be it.

a license plate number if you can, but otherwise ignore it. And take smug satisfaction in the fact that you're running. They're just getting fatter.

**KEEP AWAY FROM PAINKILLERS BEFORE YOU RUN:** If you've been feeling a little banged up or have a niggling pain that's been there for a couple days, it's tempting to take something for it so that you can get through your run okay. But this is dangerous, as it could mask the pain you actually *should* be feeling because of a developing injury. Painkillers such as aspirin, acetaminophen, and ibuprofen occasionally have their uses after a run, but never before. You don't want to go down that road.

**PAY ATTENTION TO YOUR FORM:** Don't worry too much about *how* you run. By far the more important thing is that you're doing it in the first place. But there are key things to keep in mind that will help you run smoother and easier:

- **Stay upright.** To ensure you're running tall and not slumped forward (a common mistake), visualize yourself as a puppet dangling beneath a string that is attached to the top of your head. Your head, torso, and legs should all align directly below that string as you run.
- **Face forward.** Keep your head level, eyes looking forward, and keep your face and jaw relaxed, with mouth slightly open. (You still sometimes hear that breathing through the nose is the best way. Not true! Simply breathe as you normally do.)
- **Keep shoulders down, with arms relaxed.** Don't let your shoulders "bunch up" around your ears. Keep arms bent at the elbows at around 90 degrees, and allow your hands and wrists to stay supple and slightly floppy. Allow your forearms to come across your stomach when they come forward, as opposed to straight forward and straight back.
- **Lean slightly.** It's best for your pelvis and butt to feel "tucked in" and forward, to guard against swayback. Keep your torso upright, with just a slight forward lean to help propel you forward.
- **Land gently, leave quickly.** Visualize yourself being light on your feet (hot coals,

ouch!) and lifting each foot quickly after each step. After a while, you won't need to think about it. Too much time on the ground with each foot will slow you down and make you a sluggish runner.

- **Think short, efficient steps.** Sprinting is all about taking long, powerful steps. With distance running, short and efficient is best, as it allows you to conserve energy. This also helps you land on the balls of your feet with each step, which is generally more efficient than landing too far back on your heels or too far forward on your toes.

**RUN MIDDAY IF POSSIBLE:** Businesses are way better than they used to be about providing workout facilities for employees to use at lunchtime. Take advantage of this! It provides an energizing break in the day (you'll be amazed how productive you are after lunch), it's light outside, and you'll develop the natural urge to eat a more healthful lunch after your run.

## DEAR KARA

**I've noticed that a lot of older women runners have really wrinkly faces. Does running cause this and should I be worried about it?**
Running does not cause wrinkly faces. But too much unprotected sun exposure does. Make sure that you are protected with sunscreen, even when it's cloudy. You can always wear a running hat to protect your face as well. Protection is the key here.

**JUST DO IT:** If you are a new runner, you will have lots of questions, and there are a million answers to those questions, some of them contradictory! But here's my little secret: running is very forgiving of cluelessness. You will still get a lot out of it even though you have no idea what you're doing—and none of us has any idea what we're doing when we start. In the end, just remember: one foot in front of the other, and repeat.

27

**ENJOY THOSE RUNNING GADGETS, BUT KEEP THEM IN THEIR PLACE:** This tip is similar in spirit to the previous one. Yes, there are all sorts of great technologies for runners these days, and many are simple and fun to use. Heart rate monitors, GPS watches, music devices, and crazier stuff such as cooling vests, antigravity treadmills, and hypoxic tents. But none of these things is essential to either your enjoyment of or your improvement in the sport. Some help me a little bit, and as a pro I'm looking for every safe and ethical advantage I can get. But it's training that accounts for 99 percent of my success and enjoyment of the sport.

**WALK, STRETCH, RUN:** With apologies to Elizabeth Gilbert, author of *Eat, Pray, Love,* what I mean here is it's best to be warmed up a little *before* you stretch, to ensure your muscles and tendons are ready for it. In fact, some runners wait and do their stretching after the run altogether. This is fine as long as you start running very gently, maybe with 5 minutes of walking.

**GET PLENTY OF FLUIDS:** But no need to overdo it. As long as you're drinking regularly during the day, there's no need to go crazy with water before or during running. (Drinking too much water can actually be dangerous.) Experts normally recommend the "8 x 8 rule" for the general population: eight 8-ounce glasses of fluid a day. That's fine for runners, with maybe a few extra celebratory gulps when you finish your run.

**THINK FREQUENCY, NOT DURATION:** A good starting-out habit is to just get out there for two, three, or four days out of the week, and don't worry too much about how far or long you're out there each time. Even if you only run for 10 minutes, that's fine—you did it. You want to establish the frequency habit so that you get used to that rhythm of being active for several days each week. Eventually you'll feel weird when you don't maintain that rhythm. That's when you know you're hooked on running for life.

## IT WORKS FOR ME

On really hot days I'll wear my long hair in a bun to keep it from hitting my back and getting sweaty, which keeps it from drying out.

I keep an extra pair of running socks, a running hat, and thin gloves in my car. There is nothing worse than driving somewhere to run and realizing it is colder than you thought it was.

Keep some old towels in your car. On hot days you can use them for your sweat. And if you get really dirty on a run, you can wipe yourself off or wrap them around you for the drive home.

When heading out for a long run, I always make sure to put a few tissues in my shorts waistband. There is nothing worse than being out on a run and having to wipe with a leaf!

**BE SOCIABLE:** I'll talk more about the importance of building a social running network in Chapter 3, but here I just want to say how key this is when you're starting out. Sure, in a way it's just you in the beginning. It's you taking those first steps. But very soon you'll find other runners who make it more fun. You can seek out running buddies by joining a local running club or by checking out the group runs that leave weekly from the nearby running store. If you're shy, you can let other runners come to you. And they will. And your first running buddy always leads to others.

**FIT RUNNING IN WHEN YOU CAN—EVEN IN SMALL INCREMENTS:** Time pressure can be the very thing that makes it hard to fall in love with running. If you are constantly worrying about everything you have to do that day while you're out for a run, you're really not giving running the chance it deserves. Fortunately, you can start with a very small amount of running and still get a lot out of it. So if you feel time-crunched, run for 15 minutes at a time. That's still enough to give running a chance to put a hook in you. And once it has, 15 minutes will no longer be enough!

**USE YOUR TRAINING SCHEDULE AS A GUIDE, NOT A BIBLE:** Many runners—new runners especially—are afraid to deviate from their training schedules. They think that only the specific workout written down on the calendar is the one that's going to provide the right stimulus to increase their fitness and that what you actually *feel* like doing is irrelevant—because it's not on the schedule. I disagree. Within reason, of course (you need to stick with a basic training framework), I think having fun is the most important part of training. Never be afraid to do the run you feel like doing if the one on your schedule just isn't going to cut it.

**STICK CLOSER TO THE PLAN AS YOU APPROACH RACES, HOWEVER:** If you decide to try a race one day, I would argue that's when it's smart to adhere to your training schedule, at least in the final weeks and days before the race. Those prerace workouts are key. They're specifically designed to help you run your best, so stick with the program if possible. Unless you get sick or injured, of course.

**RUN FOR REASONS THAT WORK FOR YOU:** Some people run because they think they should, but that kind of motivation is clearly not sustainable. It's best to pick a reason or reasons that really resonate. There's a woman runner here in Portland, Oregon, who was quoted as saying that she runs "half for vanity, half for sanity." I love that. Those are two great reasons to run!

**CONSIDER RUNNING FIRST THING, BEFORE THE CHAOS HITS:** The main point here is to pick a time of day to run that best suits your schedule and your biological clock. But if you're unsure when is the best time or you just don't have access to a shower at lunchtime, try for first thing in the morning. It's way easier to control this time slot than later in the day. Oh, and your fellow runners are in full agreement. A large survey recently asked runners when they normally run each day. Most common answer: 5 A.M.

**SLOW DOWN IN THE COLD (OR HEAT, OR WIND, OR RAIN):** You'll need to get used to running in all sorts of weather. Me, I love it. It's one of my favorite things about running. To me, cold winters are the most challenging, and I had a lot of those growing up in Minnesota. The main thing is to just go easy. When I go home to visit my family in Duluth for the holidays, I bundle up, strap on a pair of Yaktrax to my shoes, and head out the door. I slow down and keep my eyes peeled for black ice, but otherwise it's just a normal run.

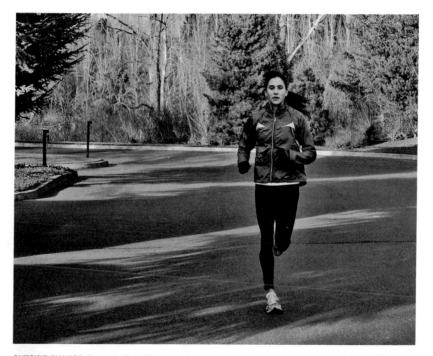

**OUTSIDE CHANCE:** Because of my Minnesota childhood, I love to get out even on the coldest days. My secret? Wearing synthetic, lightweight layers.

**GETTING STARTED**

**GET OUTSIDE WHEN YOU CAN (IT ALMOST ALWAYS BEATS THE TREADMILL):** Okay, the treadmill is great at certain times—like if it's really polluted outside, or intensely hot, or if you're traveling and staying in an unsafe part of a city. But a part of me dies a little every time I run on the treadmill. I would rather run almost anywhere than nowhere on a machine. I once ran in Croatia on tiny curbless roads packed with motorists driving like maniacs in little European cars. As bad and dangerous as it was, it was still better than running on a treadmill.

## Shoes

**BUY A DECENT PAIR OF RUNNING SHOES:** This is the one essential piece of equipment for runners, so it's important to get it right. That means going to a specialty running store where the employees are trained to get you into the right pair for you. Fit is everything with running shoes, so keep trying them on until you're satisfied with how they feel.

**SPEND THE MONEY:** Shoe experts normally recommend that you spend at least $80 on running shoes—though many cost well over $100. Of course, you can find them cheaper on the Internet or in discount stores, but in the case of the former, you don't get to try them on, which is vital. As for the latter, you never know what you're getting at a discount store, and the staff won't be trained to help you find the right pair.

**PAY ATTENTION TO SORE OR FATIGUED LOWER LEGS:** I actually don't need to keep track of how many miles I put on my shoes. I can tell my shoes are toast when I feel flat or fatigued from the knees down during two or three runs in a row. I call this "running on boards" because my feet and legs aren't getting the support they need from my shoes. Experts normally say the time-for-a-new-pair limit is about 500 miles—slightly more if you're a superefficient runner, less if you're a bigger runner or less efficient.

**BUY A SLIGHTLY BIGGER SIZE:** When buying running shoes, go for a half to a full size bigger than your normal street shoes, and simply lace them a bit more snugly. This will give your toes plenty of room so that they don't slam into the front of your shoe.

**HAVE TWO PAIRS OF SHOES AT ALL TIMES:** This way you'll always have a dry pair ready to go. They can be either the same model or different; it doesn't really matter. The one nice thing about two different types is this forces your feet and legs to deal with slightly different biomechanics. It's akin to a more well-rounded education for your brain.

**WEAR WOMEN'S RUNNING SHOES AS A RULE, BUT MEN'S VERSIONS WORK FOR SOME:** Women's running shoes tend to be designed with a slightly narrower heel and wider forefoot section, to accommodate the shape of most women's feet. But be flexible about this. If your feet are shaped such that they feel better in a men's version, go with it! (It'll be a secret only your shoe salesperson will know.)

**GO WITH A MEN'S VERSION FOR "NORMAL" COLORS:** Following the previous tip, if your feet do feel fine in a man's running shoe (and fit is the most important parameter), you'll have more color options in normal reds, blues, grays, silvers, and blacks. Women's versions tend to be pinks and pastels.

**GO SHOE SHOPPING AT THE END OF THE DAY:** It's kind of gross, but feet tend to swell slightly at the end of the day after all the normal wear and tear they get. So it's a good idea to get fitted for a new pair during this time, to give your feet and toes plenty of room inside the shoe.

33

**TRY ON BOTH SHOES WHEN YOU'RE GETTING FITTED:** Your feet can be slightly different in terms of length and shape, so be sure your shoes fit properly on both feet.

**KEEP YOUR RUNNING SHOES ONLY FOR RUNNING:** This ensures they'll stay cleaner and last longer. But it's also good to think of your running shoes as special. And, in fact, they are. They're your trusted companion and are literally with you every step of the way on your running journey.

**RECYCLE YOUR KICKS:** There are lots of great causes and charities that need used running shoes, so bypass the landfill by donating yours: Shoe donation charities include shoe4africa.org, nikereuseashoe.com, hope runs.org, and giveyoursole.com.

## DEAR KARA

**I'm new to running and I have large breasts. Will this be okay in the long term or should I pick another activity that doesn't involve so much bounce?**

As a female not blessed in that department, I feel a little silly giving you advice. But I have gotten much more endowed during my pregnancy, so I'm going to tell you what I have experienced. Don't be afraid to run because of bounce. It won't hurt you. However, it can be uncomfortable, so make sure you try on lots of sports bras until you find one that gives you proper support. You need to feel comfortable to be confident in what you are doing. A good supportive sports bra will do that for you.

# STAY SAFE OUT THERE

Running is a safe activity, but like anything that takes you out and about in the world, there are risks. Here's how to minimize them on every run:

- **Let someone know where you're going.** No need to make a big deal about it; just be in the habit of letting your significant other or housemate know your route and how long you'll be out.
- **Wear a personal ID tag on your wrist or shoelace.** You probably won't ever need it, but you may. And if you do, you will *really* need it. It's easy enough to wear it on your wrist and even easier to tie it on your shoelace so that it's there all the time. You'll find various ID types at roadid.com.
- **Bring a cell phone if you're in new territory.** Either carry it or put it in a light-weight fanny pack in case you get lost or get into any trouble.
- **Wear reflective gear in low light.** That includes overcast days and *definitely* anytime you run at night. Most running shoes and a lot of running clothes now have reflective components, but you need more. A reflective vest and hat would do it.
- **Be careful about music.** Yes, I know how you feel about your iPod, but remember to stay superalert to everything around you, including people, dogs, and vehicles. If you're running at night or somewhere secluded, turn off the music.
- **Run tall, run strong, and make eye contact.** If you do this, people will be less likely to mess with you.
- **Beware of cars pulling out on your side of the road.** If you have to run on the road, stay on the left shoulder so that you can see oncoming cars. But cars pulling out from the left may be checking traffic to *their* left as well and may fail to check right, where you are. Best to just run behind them so that if they pull out without seeing you, you'll be fine.
- **Go with a pal.** You can almost disregard all of the above—even though I don't want you to—simply by running with someone else. It's the most foolproof safety tip there is.

# The World's Simplest Beginner Running Plan

It only takes eight short weeks to become a runner. But here's the thing: you'll actually be running the very first week.

Whether you're just getting started or training for a marathon, the key is to gradually increase the amount of running you do. If you plan it right, you hardly notice the increases. Before you know it, you've reached your goal. *That* is the litmus test for a good training plan. Here is a basic but very effective plan to get you started. First, a couple of things about the plan:

- **Go three times each week:** The plan includes three workouts a week, so you'll be doing the listed workout on three separate days each week.
- **Make it convenient:** Pick any days (and times of day) that work best for your schedule, but try to be consistent with those days each week once you decide on them. Establishing a routine is vital when you're starting out.
- **Remember to rest:** Be sure you take at least one rest day between each workout day. (Easy walking or other activities are fine on rest days, just no running.)
- **Go by minutes (it's simpler):** The plan is based on minutes of running, so be sure you have a stopwatch with you.

## The Plan

**Week 1:** Run 1 minute, walk 90 seconds. Repeat eight times.

**Week 2:** Run 2 minutes, walk 1 minute. Repeat seven times.

**Week 3:** Run 4 minutes, walk 1 minute. Repeat six times.

**Week 4:** Run 6 minutes, walk 2 minutes. Repeat four times.

**Week 5:** Run 9 minutes, walk 2 minutes. Repeat three times.

**Week 6:** Run 12 minutes, walk 1 minute. Repeat three times.

**Week 7:** Run 15 minutes, walk 1 minute, run 15 minutes.

**Week 8:** Run 30 minutes continuously.

# COACH SALAZAR'S KEYS
# TO SUCCESSFUL RUNNING
# (INCLUDING MINE)

As coach of the Nike Oregon Project team I train with, Alberto Salazar works with a lot of top runners, and has done so for many years. He was a great runner himself back in the late seventies and early eighties, even holding the marathon world record at one point. After all his years in the sport, he definitely knows what makes runners successful, regardless of their ability level. These are his tips for success:

- **Be consistent:** Probably the most important strategy of all.
- **Maintain balance:** It's so important to have other things in life that matter to you more than running, even if you're an elite runner and make your living from the sport. Kara is so good about this. Her marriage, her new baby, her mother and sisters, the rest of her family—running comes after all that.
- **Hang tough:** You have to be able to absorb setbacks and stay motivated to get through them. Kara is very resilient. When things don't go well, she's good at bouncing back. She can also take a lot in workouts. She can train like crazy.
- **Take care of the big *and* little things:** If you want to keep improving, you need to care about everything that affects your running. Nutrition, cross-training, stretching, regular sleep. Everything. Sometimes neglecting something small can really have a big impact.
- **Gain all-around strength:** Physical strength counts a lot in distance running. Kara is very strong; she does not have a slight, wispy frame.
- **Stay healthy:** You can't train properly if you're not healthy or you get injured a lot.
- **Be willing to absorb pain:** To run well, you have to be able to do this. Running is not an easy sport. At the end of some of our workouts, when my runners think they're done, I'll sometimes add something unplanned. Another fast mile on the track, for instance. I do this so that my runners will learn that there's always something in the tank when they thought there wasn't. This never fazes Kara. She

is stonefaced about it and doesn't flinch. It's pretty amazing, but it's just the way she is.

# DEAR KARA

**When I run, I'm self-conscious about my body. Can you help?**

All I can say is that everyone is self-conscious about their body. I run for a living and I constantly feel self-conscious. I think, Is my cellulite showing? Are my thighs jiggling? Can everyone tell that I ate a DQ Blizzard last night and then a bag of M&Ms? I can get so insecure, but when I see other women running I always think that they look amazing. I see them out there running for their health and their piece of mind and I think they look so powerful. I can assure you that no one will judge you and others will most likely think that you are amazing to be out there running.

# CHAPTER 2

# TRAINING

A s a teenager, I did not understand the long and winding road of becoming the best runner you can truly be. Running is not a sport of instant gratification or quick results. You can improve pretty quickly in the beginning, as I did, and this early success may fool some new runners into false expectations for the future. If you stay with it, you will eventually hit a plateau of some kind. When you do, nothing can help you more than knowing that such setbacks are normal and—if you are patient and persistent—temporary. I have had many setbacks since my puberty plateau, some of them far worse than others, and I have overcome all of them. It's the same for every runner.

Even without setbacks, progress in running is a slow process. One of the keys to improving is working harder. But you can't rush this process or you will break your body down instead of building it up. You have to take small steps. If you ran 25 miles a week in training for your last race, don't jump to 50 miles a week in preparing for your next race. Your body is not ready. No matter how gifted you might be, you're human, and the human body takes its time in developing the durability needed to absorb bigger training loads. I have been a runner for twenty years and I'm still holding myself back—or at least being held back by my coach!

I ran 100 miles a week in training for my first marathon, the 2008 New York City Marathon, where I finished third. Afterward I told Alberto, "I want to run 140 miles a week! I want to do whatever it takes to win my next marathon!" Alberto would not allow it. "You're not ready," he said. And I knew he was right. Increasing my training so suddenly would have worn me out, just as my giant increase in summer running mileage wore me out before my senior cross-country season in high school.

Because I understand that developing as a runner requires small steps taken in the right order, I don't regret training in the low-key way I did under Coach Skogg. The first step in becoming the best runner you can be is laying a proper foundation, and a proper foundation is exactly what I got from Coach Skogg. More important than how much you train is how much you get out of the training you do. Throughout high school I ran about 4 miles a day, on average. This moderate level of training not only gave my body time to become stronger and better able to handle more running later, but it also encouraged me to find ways to run faster without running more.

I did this mainly by trying harder. One of the most important early lessons each runner learns is that when you think you're running as hard as you can, you're not. As you get accustomed to the pain of running hard, your tolerance for that pain increases. Everything is new for you when you are a beginning runner, and each new experience teaches you something about your body—and your mind. Discovering that some of your limitations are illusions is just one of many discoveries a new runner makes as she experiences her body's and her mind's responses to training and racing.

That's what building a foundation as a runner is really all about: gradually strengthening your body with moderate training, learning to make the most of every mile (especially by discovering how to run harder than you thought you could), soaking up experience, and getting to know your body.

Becoming a better runner is a process of continuously building on the work you have done in the past and on the fitness this work has given you. The building blocks are individual runs. Each run you do is like a brick that's added to the structure of your running fitness. Obviously this structure is not as permanent as a building. As soon as you stop running, your running fitness starts to be dismantled. But consistent training changes the body in some lasting ways. Even after a break from running, I can ramp back up to 100 miles a week pretty quickly because of lasting changes that years of running have made to my body. The foundation is always there.

Runners everywhere and at every level, from high school freshmen to world champions to masters (age forty and older) runners, use only a handful of different types of building blocks to increase their fitness. More advanced runners do longer and faster versions of these

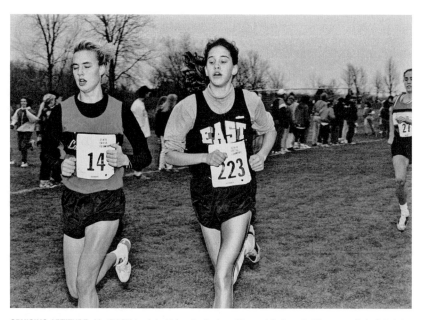

**CRUISING APTITUDE:** Me (#223) back in high school where I learned that gradual increases in both training volume and intensity are the surest way to success.

workouts, but the essential formats are the same for every runner. If you know how to do these workouts, there's really not much else you need to know about training, except how to arrange your workouts in the best way to prepare for races. Experience will teach you everything else.

The five basic types are easy runs, long runs, tempo runs, speed-work, and hills. (Of course, there's racing, too, but we'll talk about that in Chapter 7.) You'll learn about these runs and many other ins and outs (sometimes ups and downs!) of training in this chapter.

# PROVEN WAYS TO
# HELP YOU RUN FASTER
# AND EASIER

Some people, new runners especially, have a problem with the word *train*. They think it sounds too serious. "I don't train," they say. "I run." Or, "I'm a fitness runner. I don't need to train."

I understand that, but I think there's something to say for the concept of training, no matter your ability level or what you hope to gain from running. To me, training confers a level of seriousness to the endeavor, and I think that's important. Arguably, using the term means you respect what you're doing and respect yourself for doing it. It elevates things a bit, you know?

The tips and advice in this chapter are designed to help you become a better runner. I suggest you have a look through all of them and determine which ones resonate for you. Add these to your repertoire right away, as they can make an immediate impact on your training.

You'll also find some excellent cross-training tips here, as cross-training is vital to runners of all levels. It helps you burn calories, get all-around fit, and it's varied and fun. It can also make you a better runner.

To me, this chapter is the real guts of the book. After all, it's all about the training. When it comes to running, there aren't any short-cuts, but you can certainly be smarter about your training. Here are some ways to make that happen.

## I LOVE THIS QUOTE

Coming off the last turn, my thoughts changed from "One more try, one more try, one more try . . ." to "I can win! I can win! I can win!"
—Billy Mills, 10,000-meter gold medalist in the 1964 Olympics

I love this quote because Billy is explaining a thought process that we all go through when we have a breakthrough. We go from wishing to believing to doing.

**THINK *REST* DAY RATHER THAN RUNNING DAY:** Instead of saying, "I'm going to run three days this week," say, "I'm going to give myself at least three rest days this week." The ol' reverse psychology—it works!

**EACH WEEK, TRY DOING ONE SHORT, ONE LONG, AND ONE SPEEDY RUN:** This may be the simplest, most effective way to get and stay fit forever as a runner.

**SKIP A DAY:** When most runners aren't feeling well and every run seems hard, they think they're not doing enough running. But it could be you're doing too much. Or maybe work or school has been tough lately. Running can sometimes help in these instances, but other times, it's too much. Give yourself a break.

# I LOVE THIS QUOTE

Training is a case of stress management. Stress and rest, stress and rest.
—Brooks Johnson, famed U.S. sprint coach

I love this quote because it simplifies a very important principle. Without proper rest, you cannot continue to stress your body.

**START MORE SLOWLY EACH TIME OUT:** Figure out a time frame that works for you—3 minutes? 5 minutes?—and walk or jog very slowly for that period before getting into your normal training pace. This gives you time to get warmed up and can make the rest of your run feel a lot better.

**BE *SMART* ABOUT GOAL SETTING:** Having a goal or goals (a short- and a long-term one, for example) can be extremely effective in running. An effective goal can motivate you to do things you never thought possible. The best goals are called SMART goals, because they are:

45

- Specific: For example, I want to be able to run continuously for 30 minutes.
- Measurable: You can measure yourself as you run with a stopwatch. Check.
- Attainable: You are going to take six weeks to gradually work up to the 30 minutes of running, so yes, this goal is attainable. Check.
- Relevant: You care very much about being able to run for a half hour straight, so this is a relevant goal for you. Check.
- Time based: Yes, 30 minutes is time based. Check.

You can even take this SMART goal-setting method a step further by making it a SMARTER goal, which allows you to:

- Evaluate: Is it working for me? Is it keeping me motivated?
- Reevaluate: After I accomplish the goal, was it rewarding? Was it the right one for me?

**ADD A LITTLE SPEED TO MAKE RUNNING EASIER:** Okay, a bit counterintuitive here, but a regular dose of faster running will get you fitter, which will then make your regular training runs feel easier.

**ADD A LITTLE DISTANCE AS WELL:** You'll get stronger and have better endurance if you do a longer run once a week or once every two weeks. This will make your regular-length training runs easier.

**RUN HOW YOU FEEL:** Sure, you need to have a general framework for your running—three to five days a week, for example. But within that framework, do each run according to how you feel. You're feeling good today? Go harder or longer. Not so good? Do your 3-mile minimum and call it a day. This keeps your running in sync with your mind and body.

**CONSIDER RUNNING BY TIME, NOT DISTANCE (AND DEFINITELY NOT SPEED!):** This is the absolute simplest way to train. Since you can't make time go any faster, you won't be tempted to run faster. A good method is to run for half the time you've given yourself to run that day—then turn around. Simple.

**HAVE YOUR OWN KEY WORD:** Use this key word for when things get tough during a run. Or use it *before* your run, if you don't feel like heading out. Say it to yourself mantra-like. A word I used during a really tough time in my career was *fighter*. That was what resonated for me, and it worked.

**KEEP SPEEDWORK SIMPLE:** Most running experts agree that the best, fastest way to get fit is to add some regular speedwork to your program. Problem is, a lot of runners—beginners especially—are scared off by the term *speedwork*. And I admit that *speed* and *work* may well conjure up another word: *pain*. But speedwork doesn't have to be painful, it doesn't have to be complicated, and it certainly doesn't have to be done on a track (aka the Oval Torture Chamber). Rather, on your next easy run, throw in five 1-minute segments where you're running halfway between your jogging pace and your sprinting pace. It's fun, energizing, effective, and you can build up from there.

47

# I LOVE THIS QUOTE

If one can stick to the training throughout the many long years, then willpower is no longer a problem. It's raining? That doesn't matter. I am tired? That's beside the point. It's simply that I just have to.
—Emil Zatopek, three-time track gold medalist at the 1952 Olympics

I love this quote because if you can just gut through the routine long enough, it becomes second nature. This is especially true for beginners. At first you may feel as if you will never be able to stay committed to the task, but if you see yourself through it, it becomes a part of your life and ingrained in who you are.

**SEEK OUT HILLS:** I mentioned hill running in the last chapter, but it warrants further elaboration, as it is *so* effective as a training tool. As with speedwork, hills intimidate lots of runners, but they shouldn't if you use them properly. (They're almost as good as speedwork for boosting fitness.) A good way to start hillwork is to find a gently sloping hill and run five 30-second efforts up it, with a jog back down to the start after each. From there, you can increase the number of uphill efforts or the duration of each. As with speedwork, do this session no more than once a week if you're fairly new to running. Twice a week is fine for more experienced runners.

**BE WARM AND LOOSE BEFORE THE TOUGHER STUFF:** Before doing speed sessions or hills or any other higher-intensity running, run easy for at least 5 to 10 minutes to get your muscles and tendons warmed up, and your heart rate up as well. Also, look for smooth, even surfaces; keep your form fluid and controlled, start with a relatively easy speed or hill segment; do at least 5 to 10 minutes of very easy running after the tougher stuff; and take an easy or take an off-day the next day.

**HANG IN THERE DURING YOUR TEENAGE YEARS:** If you're a very young woman reading this book or if you have a young daughter or granddaughter who is a runner, here's some advice about running through puberty. It can be tough, so be patient! It certainly was for me. For a couple of years when my body was really changing fast and I was becoming a woman, my running suffered. I thought I would never get back to where I was. It took a couple of years, but I did. And you will, too. Still, I wish I had met an older runner back then to pull me aside and say, "Listen, Kara, I've been where you are, and look at me now. It's just puberty, girl!" So that's what I'm telling you now—it's just puberty.

## DEAR KARA

**Is it okay to train and race when I'm having my period? Do you do this?**

It is absolutely fine to train and race when you are having your period. Some of my best races have come right after I had my period. Train through it!

**RACE YOUR WAY INTO TOP SHAPE:** Some runners use races as their speedwork, which can actually work quite well. Sure, you have to pay a little for it, but your speed session is well marked and free of traffic, you usually have access to drinks along the way, and you get cheered for your efforts. With this alternative, who needs boring old speedwork?

**ALWAYS HAVE A FALLBACK RUN:** By this I mean a favorite training run you can depend on that's safe, easy, relatively short, convenient, and as scenic as possible. This is the run you can depend on when you don't have much time but are determined to get in a run that day. It's the run you can still get out the door for even when you really don't feel like running. It's the run you can still manage on blazing hot days or bitter cold nights. It's the run you can almost do in your sleep and often seems to take less time than you thought it would. Now that's a fallback run!

**SLOW DOWN IN THE HEAT:** Of all the tips and strategies for hot-weather running—getting extra water, wearing shades and breathable clothing, running in the morning—this arguably trumps them all. I've found that as long as I'm running slow and easy and keeping my distance down, I can run even on the hottest days. Your body is working hard to keep you cool. Help it out by slowing down. Like *way* down.

**RUN IN YOUR BARE FEET ON OCCASION:** Barefoot running is actually all the rage at the moment, and many experts believe that it's the way we were meant to run. Regardless of whether you want to jump into it with—ahem—both feet, it's a good idea to at least do it in small doses as a way to improve foot and leg strength. Be careful of sand, however, as it doesn't provide even support. It's best to start with a few easy 100-yard strides on a flat, even stretch of grass, then build up gradually from there. Pay close attention to your feet and legs along the way. They will be your guide. If you're worried about glass or other sharp objects, you can always try a minimalist shoe such as the Nike Free. It will provide protection but will still make it seem as if you're running barefoot.

**HOLD SOMETHING BACK IN WORKOUTS—ALWAYS:** Even if you are supercompetitive and are determined to reach your very best, save the 100 percent effort for the races. If you go to that "well of pain" too often, you run the risk of it drying up.

**MEET ONCE A WEEK:** You probably won't need or want to run with your training buddy every day; once a week normally works well. And early morning is probably best, before things get crazy later in the day. Oh, one more thing: meet at a neutral spot—halfway between your two houses, for example—as this assures you'll both get up on time and get out the door. (Neither of you will want to leave the other hanging.)

**EMBRACE THE POWER OF RECOVERY:** After a hard race or workout, it's so important to back off for a few days. (Make that a few *weeks* after a marathon.) This downtime gives your body and mind a chance to repair and rejuvenate themselves, which will make you stronger. If total rest drives you nuts, cross-train with cycling, swimming, yoga, or Pilates.

**JUST GO FOR A MILE:** Sometimes it's the type or length of a scheduled run that puts you off, rather than the act of running itself. If you find yourself dreading a run or doing anything but getting out the door, let yourself off the hook. Tell yourself you're just going to get in 10 minutes or an easy mile. Nine times out of ten, if not nineteen times out of twenty, once you're out there, all will be fine and you'll extend your run.

**FOLLOW THE 25 PERCENT QUALITY RULE:** The surest way to get bored with running is to run the same pace every day. Plus, in terms of fitness level, you tend to plateau pretty quickly following the "monopace" method. Better to mix in some speedy stuff each week, whereby about a quarter of your running is of a higher quality, whether that's hills, trackwork, speed pickups—basically anything that's faster than your normal running pace.

**GO EASY *AFTER* YOUR WORKOUT:** Many of us are pressed for time, but it's important to ease into *and* out of our workout. You already know that first part—some walking or very easy running along with a minute or two of positive visualization is the best way to start all your runs. But it's also important not to rush back into your day after your run. Take a few minutes to walk, stretch, talk, or just think before getting back on the treadmill of life.

51

# The Best Stretches for Runners

As a runner, you want to emphasize stretches for the legs and lower back, since that's where most of the stress occurs. What's more, the stretching method you use is probably less important than the fact that you stretch in the first place—which you should, to maintain range of motion and maybe even lower your injury risk. Static, dynamic, active-isolated, yoga—all these methods work fine, and there are many others besides.

Always remember to stretch when you're already warmed up, such as after a few minutes of walking or after your run. The following 5-minute routine should cover you nicely.

## Against the Wall

### Target: Calf and Achilles

**Stand facing a wall with one foot approximately 2 to 3 feet from the wall and the other leg extended farther back.** The rear leg should be straight, the front leg should be bent, and your hands should touch the wall. Point your feet straight ahead at all times, with your heels on the ground. Hold for 3 seconds and switch legs. Repeat 5 times. Do the exercise again, but this time bend your extended leg, which will work the lower calf.

## Hurdler Stretch

### Target: Hamstring

**Place one foot, with your leg straight, on a 2-foot-high step or a bench.** Bend your body forward and bring your head toward the leg until you feel a pull. Hold this position for 3 seconds. Switch sides. Repeat 5 times.

**BE OPEN TO—AND PATIENT WITH—NEW THINGS:** Just because you're good at one type of running (distance, for instance), doesn't mean you'll be good at everything (such as shorter, faster running). Therefore, when you try new things with your running, be prepared that not everything is going to go smoothly. Give it time. Some new training methods that

## Ankle Grab

### Target: Quadriceps

**While placing a hand on the wall or a tree for balance, use the other hand to grab your ankle.** Pull the ankle straight up behind you toward your buttocks while keeping your legs in alignment and knees together. Keeping your torso straight up and down, bring your bent knee back until you feel the pulling, hold the stretch for 3 seconds, then relax. Repeat 5 times with each leg.

## Knee Clasp

### Target: Hamstrings and Lower Back

**Lie on a firm surface.** A carpeted floor or grass is best. Bring both knees to your chest. Hold for 3 seconds. Repeat 5 times. This stretches the hamstrings and lower back. Then do the same exercise but with one leg at a time, while keeping the other leg straight.

## Chest Push-up

### Target: Abs and Lower Back

**Lie face down on the floor or ground with your legs, hips, and abdomen pressed flat onto the floor.** Place your hands on the floor beneath your shoulders. Push your chest up with your arms as far as you can go without pain and hold for 3 seconds. Repeat 5 times.

you really dislike at first will end up being your favorites, the ones you depend on most.

**LEAVE THE WATCH AT HOME:** I know a lot of runners who never leave the house without their GPS watches, which give them instant feedback

## DEAR KARA

**I've been a runner for almost thirty years and it has always kept me rail thin. The last year or so, I've started to gain weight. Not a lot yet, but I'm worried. What can I do?**

Maybe it is time to shake it up a bit. Do you lift weights? Do you do stretching exercises? Thirty years is an incredibly impressive amount of time to be dedicated to running. But it is also a long time for your body to get used to the running. It's time to change things up a bit. Add some strides to your routine, do a little backward running, lift some weights, and stretch dynamically. Shaking things up will surprise your body and get it going again.

on everything, including their real-time pace. At least once a week, run without the stopwatch or GPS. It can be liberating.

## I LOVE THIS QUOTE

Somewhere in the world someone is training when you are not.
When you race him, he will win.
—Tom Fleming's Boston Marathon training sign on his wall

I love this quote because as runners we always want to push more. As an elite runner, I am always wondering if I am doing enough. I know in my heart I am not.

**LISTEN TO STORIES:** As with listening to music while running, you need to be safe about digital books. Use them only in safe public areas during the day, or on the treadmill. Once you're sure of a safe environment, listening to books is arguably *way* better than listening to music. It's distracting—but in a good way. For one thing, music gets repetitive unless you're good about constantly downloading new stuff onto your listening device. With books, your options are endless and constantly changing. Hey, it's reading. I don't have to sell you on that!

**MAKE IT A HABIT TO FINISH STRONG:** In all your workouts, make a conscious point of starting easy so that you finish strong. If it's a speed or hill session, do that last repetition hard. If it's a long run, pick it up the last mile or so. This habit builds confidence and carries over nicely to racing. And life, for that matter.

**SET CHALLENGING RUNNING GOALS THAT YOU CAN ACCOMPLISH:** Setting a high goal is praiseworthy, but if it's too tough for you to reach, it won't do you any good. Rather, set reasonable goals that cause you to stretch a little, then keep raising your goals gradually.

## IT WORKS FOR ME

Starting and ending my run from my gym makes it much more likely that I'll follow through on my weights and stretching routines.

## Hills

**"CHIP" YOUR WAY UP HILLS:** Olympian and longtime running coach Jeff Galloway has a hill-running method that I love. It's called CHP, which stands for chest, hips, push. That is, when running uphill, keep your chest up (don't hunch over), hips forward, and push it strongly with each foot.

**RUN HILLS THE LOW-IMPACT WAY:** Hills are excellent for boosting your fitness, but downhill running can be tough on your shins and may increase

# The Best Cross-Training Activities for Runners

To become stronger, fitter, more toned—and perhaps a better runner on top of it—add one or more of these activities to your weekly running program.

## Cycling

- **How:** Extrapolate workouts from running workouts. That is, do intervals, long rides, sprints, and hills, just like you would train for running, only longer on the bike.
- **Why:** Improves endurance and leg strength (emphasize the "up" stroke for hamstring activation, which is often neglected and deficient in runners). The cyclical nature of the stroke mimics running biomechanics in a non-weight-bearing environment. Studies show that cycling can improve 10K race times by 9%, 5K by 3%, 2 mile by 1%, and boost VO2 max by 3%.

## Elliptical Training

- **How:** This is so much like running but without any pounding, as your feet never leave the pedals. So you can do pretty much all your running workouts on the elliptical.
- **Why:** Improves endurance and leg strength, burns lots of calories, and protects you from injury thanks to its "gliding" aspect.

## Inline Skating

- **How:** Find some flat ground to cruise along. Increase the workout time to get the same benefits as running.
- **Why:** A nonimpact way to strengthen all leg muscles, especially the oft-neglected glutes and hips.

your injury risk. The answer? Do hills on a treadmill, where you'll get all the benefits of going uphill without the risks of going downhill.

## Pilates/Yoga

- **How:** Find a local class at a gym or private session.
- **Why:** Improves strength, core stability, overall flexibility, and it's relaxing and fun.

## Pool Running (or Aqua Jogging)

- **How:** Mimic the same workouts run on land, now in the pool. Use a belt to add buoyancy or go without a belt to increase the intensity.
- **Why:** It's a non-weight-bearing form of exercise that improves mental and physical endurance. A study showed that pool runners who totally abstained from running for 6 weeks were able to perform the same on race day as a second group that ran for the 6 weeks.

## Strength Training

- **How:** Focus on the major muscle groups involved in running (quads, hamstrings, gluteus maximus), but don't neglect core, hip stabilizers, and upper back.
- **Why:** Research links strength training with a 4% increase in running economy (efficient use of oxygen). It may also reduce heart rate, and can improve race times from the 5K to marathon. Protects against injury by providing a solid muscular foundation.

## Swimming

- **How:** Find a local Y or health club that schedules lap swims. Or join a masters swim team that incorporates interval and distance training.
- **Why:** You get a total body workout, especially core and upper back. Improves flexibility and endurance. Gives your joints a break because it's non-weight-bearing.

57

**GET "TOWED" TO THE TOP:** Another classic hill-running tip from Jeff Galloway is to imagine a towrope attached to the middle of your chest that is pulling you to the top of the hill. I heard this one back in high school in the nineties and I know it was around long before that. The best advice—like this tip—gets passed down. Also, it's a good idea to keep your head up and eyes looking up the hill. Looking straight down toward your feet tends to chop your stride down too much, which is less efficient.

# Mental Training

**LEAVE STRESS AT THE DOOR AS YOU HEAD OUT FOR YOUR RUN:** Stress can increase muscle tension and keep you from running and breathing deeply. Have a mantra for when you head out the door: "Running starts now." Or: "Thinking stops; running starts." Your mantra will signal to your mind and body that it's time to run, so stress can go away now. (Actually that's a really good prerun mantra! "Stress, go away now.")

**DON'T EXPECT SO MUCH:** Just go out and run. Sure, every once in a while, test yourself on a challenging run or in a race. But most of the time, just run. Like when you were a kid.

**REMEMBER THAT IMPROVEMENT IN RUNNING DOESN'T ALWAYS FOLLOW A LINEAR PATH:** If you're young, you may have growing pains and your body may change, both of which can slow you down for a while. When you're fully grown, you may get sick or injured, or you may be too busy at work, or sometimes you may just be fed up with your running. All of these things can seriously derail your running. But if you're patient and diligent, and maybe just let things take their natural course, you'll come around. And the joy will return—and with it will come improvement.

**RUN FOR THE PERSONAL SATISFACTION, PERIOD:** In the 10,000 at the Beijing Olympics, I got all caught up with the idea of medaling. That become my sole focus. I got away from what had worked before, which was running for the joy of it, for the joy I got out of being good at it.

# DEAR KARA

**I just broke up with my boyfriend and the last thing I want to do is go out running. Help!**

Try to get out the door! Getting out for a run helps you to clear your head and the endorphins will make you feel better. It will help you deal with the situation better, I promise!

**TUNE IN TO THE SENSATION OF YOUR BODY IN MOTION:** Sure, iPods can be great at times, when you're not that up for running. And running with a friend or a group of runners is the best: the conversation really passes the time. But make the most of your solo runs by focusing on the essential act of running. Feel your arms and legs working perfectly together. Listen to your breathing. Revel in your movement across the earth.

**TURN FAILURE TO YOUR ADVANTAGE:** Sometimes with a race or even a workout, things don't go at all how you hoped they would. Yes, that can be depressing and even humiliating—I've been there, I know—but only give yourself a little while to wallow in that. Then take a clear-eyed look at what may have caused it and move one. If you keep a training log or running diary, review it to see what happened. Oftentimes the answer is right there in black and white.

**DETERMINE WHAT'S CAUSING SUCCESS AS WELL:** As runners, our tendency is to do intense self-examination (read: beat ourselves up) when things go bad, but we sail blindly, blissfully along when things are going well. Closely examine what's behind the good times. Chances are it's not pure luck; you're doing something right, probably several things. Your job is to figure out what they are so that you can keep doing them!

**MAKE USE OF GUILT, BUT DON'T BE DRIVEN BY IT:** Guilt isn't all bad. Sometimes it gets us out the door for a run when nothing else would. Just

59

**TRAINING**

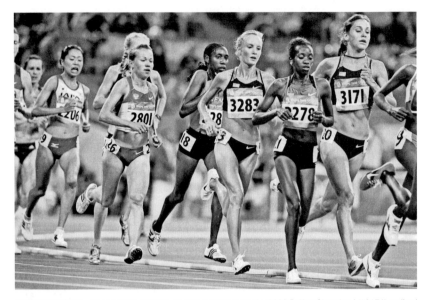

**PRECIOUS MEDAL:** After my disappointing 10,000-meter race at the 2008 Beijing Olympics, I (#3171) realized I'd become obsessed with medaling and had forgotten how to enjoy running.

don't let it become the prime mover of your running. If that starts happening, it's time to do a major rethink.

**EMBRACE THE SOLITUDE:** Running with others is great; you can share so much on a run. But maybe the best thing of all about running is the time you have by yourself, when your mind can wander. I do my best thinking while I'm running.

**BE HAPPY WITH EVERY MILE:** It doesn't matter how slow you run—you're still burning around 100 calories a mile, you're still doing all sorts of great things for your body and spirit, and you're still doing something that a very low percentage of people in this country can do: you're running.

**EMBRACE BAD-WEATHER RUNS:** Okay, running on a beautiful sunny day is pretty great, but . . . every day isn't like that, at least not in Portland, Oregon, where I live! My point is, one of the things that is so great about being a runner is the "bring it on" attitude that so many of us have. So it's raining. So it's snowing. So it's doing a little of both, with wind thrown in for good measure. That might stop the other person, but it's not going to stop *you*. And the feeling you get afterward, after running by all those people looking at you like your were nuts? Priceless.

# I LOVE THIS QUOTE

All top international athletes wake up in the morning feeling tired and go to bed feeling very tired.
—Brendan Foster, British distance runner and former world record holder

I love this quote because it humanizes elite runners to everyday runners. People think that we are superhuman, but when I am in full training, I am tired *all* of the time.

**PICK THE TOUGHER OPTION IF GIVEN A CHOICE:** You know those runs where you come to a point where there are two options for getting home? One is a flat 2 miles. The other is a hilly 2 miles. My advice? Get in the habit of taking the hilly option. Same goes for that park trail you love. There's one version that hugs the lake and stays flat. And there's the other option that's longer and takes in the hills away from the lake. They both end up in the parking lot. So my question is, once you're finished and standing in the lot, will you feel better about yourself after taking the easier route or the harder route?

**ROUND DOWN YOUR DAILY MILEAGE:** Plenty of runners "cheat" somewhat when they tally up their daily or weekly mileage. If they've done 3.7 miles, they call it 4. If they run for 19 minutes, they call it 20 in their training log. Be one of those runners that rounds *down* instead. This way you'll always have that psychological advantage—come race time or anytime—that you've actually done more than you tallied.

**BE SPECIFIC WITH YOUR POSITIVITY:** Thinking positive is such an important part of running and racing well, but I used to be pretty bad at it. My

61

thoughts in a positive-thinking session usually went like this: "I am running smoothly and powerfully. My breathing is relaxed. I wonder what I should make for dinner tonight." Then I started working with my current sport psychologist, Darren Treasure. He advises me to find and hold on to actual *evidence* that I will do well—evidence such as a great workout I did recently or a great training week leading up to a race. Evidence is the true source of confidence, and the more specific the better.

## ON THE CONTRARY

**Unlike most people, I do strength training right up until two or three days before a race.** I start backing off in intensity about two weeks out, but I do light reps right up until a few days before the race. It really helps me to feel like that muscle memory is sharp and intact.

**I don't like to be as lean as possible during heavy training periods.** For the bulk of training, I like to be about 5 pounds heavier than I'd like to be on race day. I feel like it protects me from injury and illness.

**I like to keep up my speedwork, and real speedwork, during marathon training.** If I'm training 120 miles a week and I can still knock off 200s in 30–32 seconds comfortably, just think of how easy 5:30-mile pace will feel.

**A lot of people think that to get better they need to do more mileage.** I think this can be a mistake. If you have hit a plateau, think of incorporating new training devices into your routine. Add plyometrics, core drills, weight sessions, and so on. This can often do much more for a person than more junk mileage.

## Cross-Training

**SUPPLEMENT YOUR RUNNING WITH ACTIVITIES YOU ENJOY:** Wait, isn't running enough? You ask. Followed by: How can I do more activities when it's hard enough to fit the running in? I'll provide more detailed answers, but for now the answer to that first question is . . . no, running isn't enough. To be truly fit and firm, you need to do a bit more. But don't worry—not much more! As for fitting in more exercise time, it's the same thing as running. If it's a priority, you'll find the time for it if you're smart and efficient about it. Now, as for the why . . .

**DO THE BIG THREE EACH WEEK—AND HOPEFULLY FOR THE REST OF YOUR LIFE— FOR ALL-AROUND FITNESS:** Experts recommend that for optimal health and fitness you need to do aerobic exercise, strength exercise, and flexibility exercise. Here's a quick rundown of the three:

- **Aerobic:** Generally accepted as the most important, aerobic exercises such as running raise your breathing and heart rate for an extended amount of time. Regular aerobic exercise strengthens your heart and lungs, and lowers your risk of obesity and a wide array of chronic diseases. Other examples are cycling, swimming, walking, rowing, inline skating, even gardening and yardwork. Recommended frequency: at least three to five times a week.
- **Strength:** Important for bolstering bone and muscle strength and boosting metabolism, strength exercises include lifting weights (either via free weights or machines), calisthenics (pull-ups, push-ups, etc.), yoga, Pilates, and plyometrics (bounding exercises). Recommend frequency: two to three times a week, but never on back-to-back days.
- **Flexibility:** Stretching exercises and activities such as yoga and Pilates help with your range of motion, they can decrease your injury risk, and they help you recover from injury. Recommended frequency: two times a week.

**AS YOU GET OLDER, ADD A FOURTH ACTIVITY TYPE—*BALANCE*—TO YOUR EXERCISE PLAN EACH WEEK:** If you're getting a steady dose of the first three activity types, your balance will likely be fine, but it's definitely worth paying attention to balance, especially in your sixties, seventies, and beyond, when your fall risk increases. Activities such as tai chi, balancing on one foot, and doing exercises on a wobble board can also help your running at any age, as they improve proprioception. This is

# DEAR KARA

**I've been a competitive runner since high school and now I'm thirty-eight. I think I'm starting to slow down no matter how hard I train, and it's killing me. Any advice?**

I hate to say this, but it might be time to start readjusting your goals. No one is superhuman, and we all have a time when we will start to slow down. I see thirty-eight as my last great year of racing, and then I'll have to decide if I can be happy with the performances that I can get from my body after that. There is no reason that you can't still race well and fast; you might just need to adjust your level of expectation. And remember, you are not a slacker—it is just life!

your body's ability to sense where it is in relation to the ground and where your body parts are in relation to each other.

**CROSS-TRAIN FOR ADDED CALORIE BURN:** Running tends to be the best incinerator of all (hey, that's only fair—you're working hard out there), but depending on which cross-training activities you choose, you can do some pretty serious scorching. Here's how many calories a 130-pound woman will burn in 30 minutes of activity:

| | |
|---|---|
| Running | 300+ calories |
| Elliptical training | 300+ calories |
| Pool running | 300+ calories |
| Bicyling | 236 calories |
| Swimming | 236 calories |
| Skiing | 206 calories |
| Soccer | 206 calories |
| Aerobics | 206 calories |
| Stair-climbing | 177 calories |
| Brisk walking | 118 calories |

CROSS-TRAIN FOR VARIETY: Doing a range of activities each week keeps things interesting, which of course makes it more likely that you'll keep doing them. Again, go with things you like, and keep evolving them over time. Health clubs are great places for keeping up with the latest exercise, activity, or dance craze. Go ahead and jump on the bandwagon. And keep in mind that it works well to mix activities during the same session. At the gym, start with 10 minutes on the stationary, switch to the elliptical trainer for 10 minutes, and finish up on the rowing machine for 10 minutes. I guarantee that 30 minutes will go by much faster than 30 minutes of doing only one of those three activities.

## DEAR KARA

**My butt and thighs are not as toned as I'd like them to be. Do you think running will be enough to help or should I do other toning exercises? Can you recommend any?**

Running will definitely tone things up. But as extra insurance I'd add lunges in different directions and body squats. That will tighten up your legs and butt quick!

CROSS-TRAIN SO THAT YOU HAVE A FALLBACK IF YOU CAN'T RUN FOR A BIT: Not to jinx you or anything, but there's a lot to say for not putting all your eggs in one exercise basket—namely running. If you can spread yourself around with cross-training, you gain all the benefits mentioned here, plus you'll also be better prepared to switch over to your alternates if you can't run for a while due to injury. Or if you just need a break from running, such as after a marathon or a tough few months of training, it's that much easier to switch to cross-training exclusively if you've already gained a level of comfort with it.

**CROSS-TRAIN DURING INJURY RECOVERY:** This is when lots of runners begrudgingly see the light on cross-training. A large percentage of runners who are "forced" to cross-train end up continuing it once their running injury heals! Why? Because it's fun, it's varied, you burn extra calories . . . you noticing a theme here? As for injury recovery, countless runners find that if they cross-train vigorously and consistently even if they can't run a step for several weeks, they don't lose any fitness. Some *gain* it. The key is to get your heart rate up high and keep it there for as long as you do when you're running. Good activities for this are cycling, pool running, lap swimming, stair-climbing, and elliptical training.

**CROSS-TRAIN FOR ALL-AROUND FITNESS:** Few things feel better in life than being totally fit from head to toe. As great as running is, it won't do that. Your upper body just doesn't get a lot of work during running. Nor do you gain flexibility (just the opposite!). So, to round things out, add cross-training activities that emphasize strength (especially of the upper body) and flexibility, as well as balance work if that's a concern. See "The Best Cross-Training Activities for Runners" on pages 56–57 for ideas.

**CROSS-TRAIN TO IMPROVE YOUR RUNNING:** Experts have debated the question for years: Can cross-training make you faster? Probably not (with very few exceptions) if you *replace* some of your running with cross-training. But if you *add* cross-training to the running that you already do, it seems logical that this could improve your running. After all, you're burning extra calories, you may be leaner, you're giving your heart and lungs more work, you're possibly gaining strength, and you're improving flexibility. Any one of those factors could help your running.

**DO STRENGTH TRAINING FOR YOUR LEGS AND BUTT:** A lot of women runners (men, too) think they don't need to do any strength work with their

## DEAR KARA

**I have this little stomach-paunch thingy that just will not go away. It drives me crazy. Can you recommend an exercise that will get rid of it?**

Stomachs are tough. And, of course, everyone's body is different. I'd look at diet and exercise to see if there is something more you can do. Do you eat enough protein? Too much sugar? Do you do core exercises, more than just sit-ups? If you are doing everything right and you still have a little stomach, it could just be life. We all have something about our body that we don't like and that we notice, but no one else does. Your stomach could be just that!

legs and backside because running does it for them. That's partly true, but not entirely. Running is great for the legs and butt. Few things are better at keeping them strong, toned, and shapely. But running also taxes the lower body in ways that can break it down and cause injury, which is where strength training comes in. Good basic exercises like half squats, toe raises, lunges, and leg curls will all help gird your legs so that they can better withstand the stresses of running. Strengthening your quads (upper front thigh muscles), to take one example, is vital for proper knee functioning. See "The Best Strength Program for Runners" on pages 70–75.

**WORK THE UPPER BODY FOR STRENGTH, TONE, AND CONFIDENCE:** As I mentioned, running doesn't do a lot for the upper body besides helping to keep it slim (as it does your entire body). You need strength work for this. Yoga and Pilates are both excellent for strengthening your upper body, as is weightlifting with either dumbbells or on weight machines. This way you'll have the sleek, toned legs from running along with the toned and sexy arms, shoulders, and chest from strength training. Confidence!

## DEAR KARA

**I want to do strength training for my core, arms, and shoulders, but I'm worried about getting too muscled. Any advice?**
This is something many women worry about, but unless you are maxing out at the gym multiple times a week, the odds are very slim that you will get too muscled. If you are really worried about it, do less weight and higher reps. This will lean you out, not bulk you up.

**BE HARD-CORE:** The so-called core muscles of the stomach, lower back, buttocks, and upper legs are absolutely key to successful, injury-free running. It's where so much of your power comes from during each running stride. Your core muscles help lift your leg forward and drive it back with each step. During running, your core muscles also connect your legs with the power you're creating with your arm swing, which helps propel you forward. Think of this visual next time you're wondering if you need to do core work: without a strong core, your legs will "dangle" beneath you, puppet-like and disconnected from the rest of your body.

## I LOVE THIS QUOTE

You must always realize one thing. In every little village in the world there are great potential champions who only need motivation, development, and good exercise evaluation.
—Arthur Lydiard, famed New Zealand running coach

I love this quote because I love the idea that it doesn't matter where you come from, you have the potential to be great.

**GAIN AMAZING BENEFITS FROM YOGA:** You already know how great yoga is for building strength and flexibility. Recent research has found that it does an incredible number of other things as well, including improve balance, decrease pain levels in seniors, reduce menopausal symptoms, and boost energy levels. What's more, it could play a key role in your weight-control efforts, thanks to its ability to reduce stress. Researchers have found that lowering your stress can decrease high-fat and high-sugar food cravings.

**ADD PLYOMETRICS TO YOUR PROGRAM:** Plyometrics is a jumping-based form of exercise that helps develop a more powerful and efficient running stride. I never had a good finishing kick until I started doing plyometrics; now I feel like I have an extra gear when I need it. Plyometrics is simple. Skip on one leg, then switch legs. Or jump forward for distance on one leg or two. Or skip with an exaggerated bounce. Do these a couple times per week after your runs or even during your runs. For example, switch from running normally to skipping for height for 30 seconds, jog a little more, then hop on your right leg for 20 steps, then your left leg for 20 steps. Simple as that.

**BOLSTER YOUR UPPER BODY TO CONTROL YOUR ARM SWING:** A strong upper body means you'll be less likely to swing your arms too far across your chest with each running stride. This creates wasteful "twisting" and doesn't propel you forward efficiently. So think about running tall (no slouching!), squared shoulders pointing forward, and good, active, front-to-back arm swing. Working with 3-pound dumbells is a simple way to improve your upper body running form.

69

# The Best Strength Program for Runners

*Devised by my strength-training coach, Tony Salazar (Alberto's son), the following program will help make you a better, stronger runner. And you only need to do two sessions a week, each lasting well under an hour.*

Women runners aren't as good as their male counterparts about doing regular strength training, which is too bad, because it offers an important array of benefits. A well-designed program will help you build overall strength, improve your muscle tone, burn more calories, and lower your injury risk. Women often give one of two reasons (sometimes both!) for not doing strength work: they don't want to bulk up, and it's too boring.

The first one simply isn't true. Men sometimes bulk up, which is not always the best thing for their running, but women? "It almost never happens," says Salazar. "Improved muscle tone, sure. But too many muscles? Almost never."

As for the "too boring" excuse, that's where Salazar's plan can help, because there's lots of variation, yet the exercises are simple to learn and execute. You do just two sessions a week—and remember, always separate them by at least one to two days—and each session involves a completely different set of eight exercises. Result: plenty of variation, and you really work the whole body.

Before getting to the exercise descriptions, here are four important points:

1.  **Lower the reps, raise the weight.** Each week for 4 weeks, you'll be lowering the repetitions you do with each exercise but increasing the weight. But always aim for three sets of each exercise. Here's how it looks:

    **Week 1:** 3 sets of 12
    **Week 2:** 3 sets of 10
    **Week 3:** 3 sets of 8
    **Week 4:** 3 sets of 6
    **Week 5:** Off

*Note:* Take every fifth week off completely, then return to week 1 (i.e., 3 sets of 12) but with gradually heavier weight amounts.

2.  **Remember your rest:** Rest at least 60 seconds between each set. You can do light stretching during this time.

3.  **Don't strain:** Be sure you can get through every rep without straining or losing form. If necessary, drop down in weight.

4.  **Start easy if you're new to lifting:** If you're a novice, do one set of 10 reps for each exercise for 2 full weeks *before* starting this program.

## First Session Each Week

### Exercise 1: Barbell Squat

**Keep shoulders back and chest out.** Feet shoulder width apart. Sit back and down until thighs are parallel to the floor. Pause for a split second, then stand up. Keep chest and eyes up during the entire lift. Sit back so that your knees are never going farther forward than your feet. Don't let your knees cave in at all; keep them directly above your feet the entire time. Push through your heels.

### Exercise 2: Dumbbell Incline Press

**Bench should be at approximately a 45-degree angle.** With dumbbells just outside of your shoulders, push them up until your arms lock above your head. Lower back toward your shoulders and pause for a moment before repeating. Reach to the ceiling, and control the weight on the way down.

### Exercise 3: One-Leg Dumbbell Russian Deadlift

**With dumbbell in right hand, balance on your left foot.** Keep slight (10-degree) bend in left knee. In a smooth motion, bring dumbbell down your left thigh/shin until it reaches midshin. Hold for a second, then raise back up. Attempt to keep right leg in a straight line with your back. Therefore, the leg will be straight out while dumbbell is at the bottom of the lift. Repeat with dumbbell in left hand while balancing on right foot. Keep your glutes tight and the weight close to your lead leg the entire time.

71

### Exercise 4: Pull-ups

**With palms facing away from body, grip the pull-up bar with hands outside of shoulders.** In a slow, controlled motion, pull your body upward until your chin is above the bar. Slowly lower your body back down and repeat. If this lift is too difficult to complete without assistance, you can have someone hold your feet and provide assistance. Don't cheat—go all the way down.

### Exercise 5: Dumbbell Step-up

**Holding a dumbbell in both hands, use a bench/box, which can be up to knee height.** The higher the box, the harder the lift. Firmly plant your lead foot onto the bench/box and stand up until your front leg is straight. Slowly lower your back leg back to the floor. Switch legs and repeat. Don't push off your down leg; instead, step off your lead leg.

### Exercise 6: Tri-Pushdown

**Using a cable machine, set up bar so that it rests at chest level.** Keeping elbows pinned to your sides, lock arms out at the bottom. Let bar come back to midchest and push down again. Don't cheat by using momentum; feel it only in your triceps.

### Exercise 7: Back Extension

**Keep your back straight the entire lift.** While bending at the hips, lower your shoulders toward the ground. Raise back up. Keep good form; hips to shoulders should be a straight line.

### Exercise 8: Crunches

**With knees bent at right angles, only come up enough that your shoulder blades come off the floor.** Keep head in line with torso; don't "nod" forward or otherwise put strain on your neck. Raise up faster; lower down slower.

## Second Session Each Week

### Exercise 1: One-Leg Squat

**Hold dumbbells in each hand.** With back foot resting on a bench, bring your front foot out far enough so that when you are in down position your knee is not farther forward than your foot. With chest straight up, bend your front leg until your thigh is as close to parallel as possible. Raise back up to starting position. Try to get your front thigh to parallel. Keep your front foot pointed straight forward.

### Exercise 2: Dumbbell Bench Press
**Same as Dumbbell Incline Press,** but with flat bench.

### Exercise 3: Russian Dead Lift
**Hold a barbell.** While maintaining a 10-degree bend in knees, slowly lower the weight down your thighs until you reach midshin level. Keep your back as straight as possible. Stand back up using the same path as going down. Keep your back tight; no bending. The bar should almost touch your shins the whole way down.

### Exercise 4: Chin-ups
**Same as Pull-ups,** but with palms facing in.

### Exercise 5: Dumbbell Lunge
**Hold a dumbbell in each hand.** Take a big step out, and while keeping a slight bend in back leg, lower your body until back knee is almost hitting the ground. Push off front leg and stand back up. Push all the way back to the starting position, not halfway.

### Exercise 6: Dumbbell Bicep Curl
**With a dumbbell in each hand, keep elbows pinned to your side and curl the dumbbells up toward your shoulders.** Don't swing the weight; lift it with your biceps. Don't cheat by using momentum; feel it only in your biceps.

### Exercise 7: Superman
**Lie face down on the floor.** In a smooth motion, raise both feet and hands off the floor. Hold for a pause and repeat. Don't swing or bounce off the floor.

### Exercise 8: Medicine Ball Twist
**Lie on the floor with feet off the ground and knees bent.** Holding a medicine ball/dumbbell in your hands, rotate it in a half circle from the outside of one hip to the other while keeping your feet off the ground. Don't bounce the weight off the ground; control it.

73

# Important Modifications for Pregnant Runners

After getting your doctor's permission, it is safe for you to do this strength program, with a few key changes. Always remember:

1. **Never** hold your breath. If the weight is so heavy that it requires you to hold your breath, then you need to lighten the load.
2. **Never** strain to lift a weight. You should always choose a weight that allows your muscles to fatigue, but not so heavy that you have to really strain to lift it.
3. **Never** perform a lift while flat on your back.

Also, be sure to make these important exercise modifications to the two sessions:

*For the first session of the week,* take out the Dumbbell Step-up, the Back Extension, and the Crunches, and add the Seated Leg Curl and the Plank. Here's how to do these two replacements:

## Exercise 5: Seated Leg Curl

**Sitting (depending on the machine you use), start with both legs extended.** Without letting your back arch, bend your knees until your lower legs form a 90-degree angle with your upper legs. Hold for 2 seconds, then return to the starting position.

## Exercise 7: Plank

**Lie face down with body in a straight line, with elbows and feet supporting your weight.** Hold this position for 30 to 60 seconds.

*For the second session of the week,* take out the Dumbbell Lunge, the Superman, and the Medicine Ball Twist, and add the Leg Extension and Plank Raises. Here's how to do the two replacements:

### Exercise 5: Leg Extension

Sitting on a leg-extension machine with both legs bent at 90 degrees, extend both legs until they're nearly straight (no need to "lock" your knees). Hold for a pause, then slowly release back down to the 90-degree starting position.

### Exercise 7: Plank Raises

Assume plank position. Raise right hand and left leg straight out, hold for a pause, and bring back. Repeat with opposite hand/foot.

# DEAR KARA

I don't have a lot of time to do any exercise other than running, but I feel like I should be fitter and more well rounded physically. What activity do you think is the best complement to running that would boost my all-around fitness?

I think that a simple weight program complements running excellently and will really improve your physicality. You don't have to do a lot, but some core moves a few times a week in the weight room would fit perfectly with your running routine.

# CHAPTER 3

# SOCIAL RUNNING: BUILDING YOUR SUPPORT NETWORK

I am a very social runner. Except for the few weeks before a big race, I depend heavily on a network that includes my coach and others on my support team, friends, and my husband. This network isn't important just because I'm a professional runner. If anything, it may be even more important if you're not a professional. A network can support you, teach you, lessen the blow of your failures, and share in your successes—whether that is finishing your first 5-mile training run or completing your first race.

I have had three coaches. They could not be more unlike one another, but I've had great experiences with all of them.

Coach Skogg at Duluth East High School did not have a lot of knowledge, but he more than made up for that with his warm way of relating to his runners and his deep concern for our best interests.

Mark Wetmore at Colorado was not the kind of guy who gave bear hugs to his runners, but he knew what he was doing and he instilled total

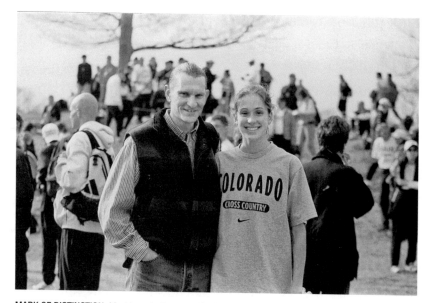

**MARK OF DISTINCTION:** Most important, you need to be able to trust your coach. I had that trust with my college coach, Mark Wetmore.

faith in all of his runners. Mark has a distinct, precise method that never changes and has produced countless champions.

My current coach, Alberto Salazar, is unique in a different way. Alberto has an uncanny ability to make runners believe in themselves. Unlike Mark, he changes things. He is willing to experiment and is not afraid to say, "I don't know," when he doesn't know. But unlike both Mark Wetmore and Coach Skogg, Alberto was once among the best runners in the world, and when he tells me that I can be one of the best, I believe him!

## I LOVE THIS QUOTE

There are three things you don't bet against. They are taxes, death—and Alberto.

> —Bill Squires, Boston-based distance coach, on Alberto Salazar

**SOCIAL RUNNING: BUILDING YOUR SUPPORT NETWORK**

I love this quote because it reminds me that my lovable and nurturing coach used to be an animal on the racing scene.

The one similarity in my relationships with all of my coaches is trust. Despite their different styles, I trusted Coach Skogg, I trusted Mark Wetmore, and I trust Alberto. Trust is a gut feeling. You cannot predict who you will and won't have faith in. Personal recommendations, track records of success, credentials, and sensible training systems are good things to consider when choosing a coach. But the feeling of trust should be the deciding factor. Trust that feeling!

Even though I've always run in team environments with lots of runners almost always around me, I've tended to have a favorite running buddy at any given time. In high school it was Amy Hill. In college it was Molly Austin. In Portland it has been Amy Yoder-Begley. I'm not sure why I've fallen into this pattern. Maybe it's because it is hard to find someone who has both personal and running compatibility with me. Or perhaps I know instinctively that my running benefits the most when I share intense competition and support with another woman.

Recently I had a very special temporary training partner: Paula Radcliffe. I was terrified when I first heard that Paula had come to Portland from England to train for a while—and that she wanted to train with me. I am in awe of Paula. Who isn't? The woman ran a 2:15 marathon. No other woman has run within three minutes of that time. I was scared that if I ran with Paula, she would destroy my confidence for all time—not because she wanted to but because she couldn't help it.

However, because I admire Paula so much, I was also excited about the opportunity to run with her, so I did. And, as I might have predicted, I don't regret it. Running with Paula was amazing. She has an incredible life. Most of Paula's American fans have no idea how popular she is in the United Kingdom. She's at the same level as David

Beckham, the soccer player. I loved hearing her stories, and I heard lots of them. When we ran together, we talked nonstop, except when we were running too hard to talk.

Although we talked about a lot of things other than running, we also talked a lot about running. We shared stories about past races and looked forward to future races and goals. One time I shared with Paula my dream of running a 2:18 marathon, which would be an American record. She told me she believed I could do it. That means a lot to me.

If you keep running long enough, you will sooner or later find running buddies that are as perfect for you as my best running buddies have been for me—if running buddies are your thing. The best places to find them are in the running groups that meet at many local running specialty shops, in running clubs, and at competitive track and road racing clubs. These different kinds of groups can help you run better and with more enjoyment, even if you don't use them to find individual running buddies.

It's important to find a group that matches your needs. If you are a noncompetitive beginner, you will probably feel most comfortable in a beginner-oriented, charity-based club like the Leukemia and Lymphoma Society Team in Training. If you're fast and are serious about getting even faster, you might be happiest on a racing-focused team that has performance standards for new members.

My husband is not a great running partner for me. Sure, we get along well and enjoy spending time together, but he's just too fast for me! I'm a world-class female runner. He's a world-class male runner. There's a pretty big difference.

Although we can't do entire training runs together, we find lots of other ways to be together as runners. All of the members of our team do pretty extensive warm-ups with light jogging, stretching, and drills, and Adam and I do these together when we can. Sometimes we share the same track for workouts, and while we don't do the same workouts, we can at least watch and encourage each other. I like to watch and

79

encourage Adam in some of his harder workouts even when I'm not running, and he does the same for me. We frequently do our stretching, strength training, and cross-training together as well.

Naturally, we cheer each other on in races. Sometimes Adam does a lot more than spectate. In 2009 I ran a big half marathon in Chicago. Adam was at the starting line to wish me good luck. When I got to the 1-mile mark, he was waiting there to give me my split time. He had run the whole first mile on the sidewalk faster than I had! But he didn't stop there. He kept going for almost the whole race—sprinting ahead, dodging spectators, shouting encouragement, taking shortcuts where he could, and giving me pace information. Adam is kind of crazy sometimes, but in a good way!

I get more nervous before Adam's races than I get before my own. It's unpleasant, but that's the price you pay for loving someone so much that his success is as important to you as your success. The joy of being able to share in Adam's successes makes that price well worth paying. And, of course, it comes right back to me. His support helps

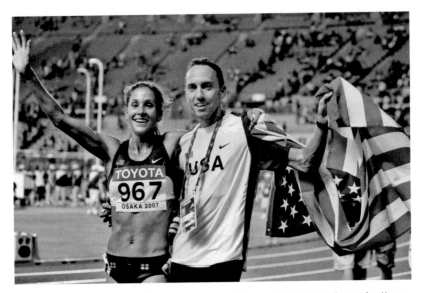

**JOINT VENTURE:** Besides being an elite runner himself, my husband, Adam, is my number one fan. Here we celebrate my bronze medal finish in the 10,000 meters at the 2007 World Championships.

me succeed and makes my achievements more satisfying, because I have someone to share them with.

There are many practical benefits to being married to another runner. Most competitive runners are prone to doing too much: running hard when we need to rest, ignoring aches and pains that should not be ignored, and that sort of stuff. Adam and I help each other avoid making stupid mistakes that we would surely make without a knowledgeable and caring partner watching out for us. We also talk each other through the self-doubt that creeps up when one of us is not running well, the frustration that comes with being injured, and other negative emotional experiences that are common in the life of every runner.

Each relationship is unique. There is no blueprint for happy relationships. Every couple has to work out their own dynamics in terms of how they communicate, how they support each other, and even how they share responsibilities. It's the same for the running element in running couples. You can't force it to work a certain way, just as Adam and I can't force ourselves to do whole runs together. But as they say, love will find a way. If you and your boyfriend, partner, or spouse allow yourselves to be led by your love for each other and your passion for running, you will find a way to share your running lives that works for both of you, even if your recipe is a little different from someone else's.

My network has been and always will be there for me. I never would have gotten as far without that constant support. I'm sure the same will happen for you. Now for some advice on building your own support network.

81

# BEST WAYS THAT COACHES, RUNNING CLUBS, TRAINING PARTNERS, OR SIGNIFICANT OTHERS CAN HELP YOU BECOME A BETTER RUNNER

Runners were linking up, chatting, sharing, gossiping, and supporting one another long before Facebook and Twitter came along. Despite that old "loneliness of the long-distance runner" rap we've lived with for too long, we tend to be a gregarious bunch and have been since Day One. Especially women runners. Us girls never bought into solitary suffering.

But I'm not saying we're a bunch of unserious gadflies, either. We run as hard as the guys, but we understand that there is strength in community. That with a little help from our friends and mentors, we'll become better runners and enjoy it more along the way. Even the lows (we all have them) won't be so low when you have a support network in place.

Looking for a coach to give you some weekly guidance? You want to join a running club, but you're worried the members are all too serious? Looking for a training partner who is totally compatible with you? The following tips for building a social running network will help with these concerns—and many more besides.

83

**JOIN THE CLUB:** Running clubs aren't for everyone, but from my experience, they're a hoot. Almost without exception, you'll find club people to be fun, optimistic, smart, and well educated, which, no surprise, is why lots of women join them to meet great guys. Here's another thing: Don't think that everyone in a running club is going to be faster than you. Not true! Slowpokes join, too, for the fun and camaraderie. It's easy to find a club near you. Just check with the umbrella organization Road Runners Club of America at rrca.org.

**QUIT IF IT DOESN'T WORK:** If the running club thing doesn't suit you, no big deal. It's no reflection on you whatsoever.

**BE OPEN TO A MENTOR:** Runners are famous for sharing advice—even when you don't want it! Seriously, lots of runners don't want a coach for whatever reason, and for those people, a mentor sometimes works way better. This is the most natural way to go for beginners. Mentoring happens all the time in running. Experienced runners share wisdom with newer runners, who later pass it on to the next wave of beginners, and so on. You may find you'll get all the guidance you need from a mentor or mentors. The surest way to find one? Join some kind of a running group—whether that's a loose group of training friends, a running club, or the group that meets weekly at the local running store.

## I LOVE THIS QUOTE

I was too embarrassed to be another fat guy in new running shoes and sweats, so we'd go out at night with a flashlight. . . . I found out that runners weren't judgmental."
—George "Norm" Wendt, actor, *Cheers*

I love this quote because I love seeing people run—people of all shapes and sizes. Runners aren't judgmental; we are proud of anyone who joins us.

**SEEK OUT GROUP THERAPY:** Again, running groups can be totally informal—a bunch of friends who meet for a run at the park every Sunday morning, for instance. Or they can be more formal, like the team I'm part of at the Nike Oregon Project. Or anything in between. But there's just something about running in groups that makes everyone better. Being part of a group can also make the running experience richer and more enjoyable. I think the two are connected, actually. Running in a group makes you run better because it makes the training process more fun.

## DEAR KARA

**There's a really cute guy in my running club who I like, but I'm faster than him and worried he'll resent that. What should I do?**

Don't hesitate to pass him. If it turns him off that you are faster, he's probably not a guy you want to be with anyway. But you might be surprised—it might impress him!

**FIND THAT SOMEONE SPECIAL:** Sometimes the best group of all consists of you and one other person. The great Ethiopian runner Kenenisa Bekele only ever runs with one other person: his brother, Tariku. He says he is comfortable running with his brother and uncomfortable running with anyone else.

**CONSIDER COMPATIBILITY:** Finding the right training partner is sometimes tougher than you might think, so it's important to think it through before you make a commitment. Everyone wants something slightly different in a partner. For you it may be someone who:

- is slightly faster than you
- is slightly slower than you
- is more sociable on the run than you

- gets up easier in the morning (you know she'll be there)
- doesn't mind running slow all the time
- is a good listener
- always tells it like it is
- is game for anything

And so on. Be patient—you'll find that person eventually. When you do, hold on tight to him or her.

**KNOW WHEN TO GO IT ALONE:** Even if you're a diehard group runner, there may be times when it's best to do your runs on your own. When you're returning from injury could be one of those times, as you're more likely to do exactly what you need to do, rather than getting pulled along by others. For the last five or six weeks before a big race, I'll tend to do more workouts by myself that are tailored to the particular distance I'll be racing. The same thing may apply to you. If you're getting ready for a hilly race, for instance, you may want to put in some solo time on your favorite hilly course.

**BENEFIT FROM YOUR OWN COACH:** You can certainly find one via the Internet (search "how to find a running coach"), but this may be a case where it's best to look the old-fashioned way. You can call the athletics department of a local university and ask to speak to the track or cross-country coach. Oftentimes these people (many of them have loads of experience) do some coaching on the side, or if not, they're usually in touch with the local scene. Or ask at your local running store. If the employees don't coach themselves, they'll know locals who do. Running clubs are another great source for information. Larger clubs sometimes have their own coaches and will meet for group workouts under that person's direction. Finally, if you don't think you need someone on-site, there are plenty of experienced, well-trained online coaches who can send you workouts, exchange ideas via e-mail, and generally provide guidance.

RUN WITH OTHERS—FOR CHARITY: Especially if you're a beginner, the best running group of all may be a charity-based outfit like the Leukemia and Lymphoma Society Team in Training. For your pledge to raise a certain amount of money for the charity, you get a coach and willing training partners, plus an energizing boost from helping out with a great cause. Search on the computer under "running for charity" for all sorts of charity options in your area.

# DEAR KARA

It sometimes annoys me that my fellow women runners are generally so much more public-spirited than men about raising money for charities. The women in my club raise way more than the guys, for instance. Why is this?

I don't know why this is, but I think it is great. A woman might not think about participating in a road race until she knows that it is for charity. If her wanting to help out a good cause gets her out the door and running on the pavement, then I think that is a beautiful thing.

# DEAR KARA

I've never raised any money for a running-related charity. Most of the women in my running club have. This is starting to bother me. Should I feel guilty?

No, you should not feel guilty. Unless something comes up that you are passionate about, don't feel like you have to raise money for a charity. People run for many different reasons, and it sounds like yours is centered more around yourself than raising money. There is nothing wrong with either reason. Don't feel bad.

**RUN WITH MEN:** Women tend to have female training partners and men tend to have male training partners. This is fine, of course, but there's something to be said for running with guys. Guys tend to bring a different perspective to things, and running is such a great time for conversation. Because everyone is relaxed and cruising along, tongues loosen, and you'll be amazed at all the topics you'll cover. Also, guys can sometimes push you to another level where you wouldn't normally go yourself. This is a great way to get faster.

## DEAR KARA

**I want to look hot (not temperature-wise!) when I run. Any tips?**
It's true that if you feel good, you'll look good. So wear clothes that you feel are flattering; wear you hair in a manner that is functional but attractive. You will look hot every time you head out to run.

**USE THE MAP MY RUN (MAPMYRUN.COM) SITE TO FIND NEW RUNNING ROUTES:** This site is great and it's really easy to use. Whether you're home, at work or college, or traveling, simply put in your starting location, then search for runner-tested routes that others have done in your area. You get all sorts of choices. You can put in various preferences, including distance and terrain. The maps are easy to read and printable.

**PACE A SLOWER FRIEND IN A RACE:** This can be so rewarding! Try to be quietly, optimistically supportive, as there's nothing worse than being paced by someone who is not having any trouble keeping the pace and isn't shy about showing it. And *always* let your friend cross the finish line first.

**RUN WHILE FAMILY MEMBERS CYCLE ALONGSIDE:** If they don't like to run or aren't in shape for it, have family members join you on occasion on a bike. One nice benefit: after the run, invariably they'll be amazed at how fit you are!

**TAKE YOUR FAMILY ON A RACE VACATION:** It's a lot of fun to travel to a race with family. This way they get an inside look at the excitement and anxiety of it, and you can share the experience with one another. Have them tag along to the race and race-number pickup, which is always so exciting. At the same time, don't feel bad about taking time to be by yourself if you need to run a few relaxing miles or want to chill back in the hotel room. They'll understand! If possible, build in some family fun and recovery days after the race when you won't be distracted or nervous, and everyone can relax and enjoy a new place.

**VOLUNTEER AT A LOCAL RACE:** It's fun, rewarding, and such a nice thing to give back to the sport that you love. Just call or e-mail the race contact number at least a month beforehand and ask what they need most.

# I LOVE THIS QUOTE

Great is the victory, but the friendship of all is greater.
—Emil Zatopek, Boston-based distance coach

I love this quote because the friendships I have made in running are the greatest of my life. And long after I am an elite racer, those friendships will continue.

**BUILD THE WIDEST SUPPORT NETWORK YOU CAN MANAGE:** Running is not always the easiest thing to want to do, and if it's not fun or you have only one partner, you're likely to be struggling. Approach groups from different places: your work, your family, your children's school, the gym, the local community, anywhere. You need to increase the opportunities that will make you run. If you have more options, you will have more fun, more experiences, and more likelihood of running.

**USE THE RUN AS SOCIAL TIME:** See runs as an opportunity to catch up with friends. It doesn't have to be dinner, drinks, or coffee. Get used to the social opportunities running provides. If you enjoy talking, start running and talking. Avoid trying to run faster or listening to your iPod. Just enjoy meeting your friends over a run. Have fun talking about your families, friends, TV, philosophy, anything.

## DEAR KARA

**I've been hoping to meet a guy at a road race (better than at a bar!), but so far it hasn't happened. Any strategy you can recommend?**
If you see someone who seems interesting, compliment him on his race, his stride, something like that. If you get a good response back from him, then continue on with some conversation. If not, don't despair! There are loads of men around waiting to be found!

**USE THIS NETWORK TO SUIT DIFFERENT OCCASIONS:** Sometimes you may want to push yourself, so organize a run with friends from the gym or the annoying person who always wants to be slightly ahead. Sometimes you may want a casual run, so call your friends around the corner. Consider what you want and need and what the personalities of the different groups are.

**BE PROACTIVE AND CLEVER:** Organize a run to start and finish at the nicest coffee shop in town. Organize a pizza party or barbecue for after the run. Organize a run in exciting places—the woods, the beach, the hills—and really explore the environment. Make it as exciting and invigorating as possible.

**RUN TO SOCIAL ENGAGEMENTS:** If you're meeting your friends in town, run there. If you're meeting your family on Sunday afternoon in the park, get your husband to drive while you run. Just make sure you're comfortable in your running gear or that you can get changed easily. The network doesn't have to be people you run with; it can be the reward for the run.

## DEAR KARA

**I'm a little embarrassed about sweating so much when I run. How do you deal with this?**

I am a sweater! I can't help it—the harder I run the more I sweat. I used to be so embarrassed, but I've just stopped worrying about it. Everyone is different, and some of us sweat more than others. Think of it this way: the more you sweat, the more efficient your body is at cooling itself.

**PLAY GAMES WHILE YOU RUN:** Take turns to lead. You have to go wherever your friends choose to go. You have to go at their pace. You have to go for however long they say. Play chase! Run the odd race to the nearest tree. Watch the weather, wait for rain, and then go running. Run through the puddles with your friends. Sing Lady Gaga or Kanye West at the top of your voices. Make it as fun as possible.

## What to Look for in a Coach

Having a coach is not just for elite runners; it's for everyone. In fact, it may be the best thing you ever did for your running. That said, it's important to find the right one for you. Here are some key points to consider when looking for a coach:

**YOU ARE THE EXPERT, NOT YOUR COACH:** An effective coach will understand that no one can know your body and your responses to training better

91

than you. A coach who is willing to learn from you is a coach who will be better at adjusting your training to meet your changing needs, reactions, and goals.

**RUNNING SHOULD BE JUST ONE ASPECT OF YOUR LIFE:** A coach who asks you to do nothing else but eat, sleep, and train is probably unaware of how easy it is for runners to overtrain, become obsessed, and possibly burn out. This type of coach is often looking for quick results, whereas you want a coach who recognizes that healthy improvement takes years of consistent work framed within a balanced lifestyle.

**PERFORMANCE IS A HOLISTIC PROCESS:** Some coaches are obsessed with their training plans and believe they can write the perfect workout. These are coaches who only focus on the X's and O's of running. But running well involves more than putting in the work. A good coach should know that you also need to feel happy, healthy, and confident to run well.

## I LOVE THIS QUOTE

Confidence is the most important quality in all athlete–coach relationships.
—Franz Stampfl, famed Austrian middle-distance coach

I love this quote because it rings so true. I have had three coaches who have had completely different coaching philosophies. Yet I have been successful under all of them because I believed in them.

**COMMUNICATION AND LISTENING ARE KEY:** A coach who is genuinely interested in your growth and development as a runner is going to ask questions more often than he or she gives directions and will listen to what you say. A coach can only be effective if he or she has lots of information about you.

**LOOK FOR A LIFELONG LEARNER:** When considering working with a coach, ask him or her what new ideas, theories, or approaches to training he or she has adopted lately. Also ask what books, magazines, or sport science journals he or she regularly reads. An effective coach will be curious and interested in learning, which is exactly the kind of person you want to trust with your development as a runner.

**NEVER IGNORE RESULTS:** Look at how other athletes who have worked with this coach fared. Did they enjoy a long and prosperous career or were they constantly injured? Similar to lawyers, plumbers, or doctors, there are some coaches who get better results than others. Do your homework, just as you would when selecting any other professional to work for you, and do not feel shy to interview a prospective coach or ask for a résumé or a list of references.

**BE CLEAR ABOUT FINANCIAL CONDITIONS:** Many coaches charge the runners they work with a fee for service. Be sure to discuss this from the start so that everyone is clear about the price and the terms. Also, what if you win some prize money? Regardless if it is likely to be a large payday or just $100 from a local road race, discuss up front whether the coach will receive any percentage of your winnings.

# CHAPTER 4

# STAYING INJURY-FREE

You might say I've had a little experience in this area, and yes, I could go on about it. But I won't. As a cautionary tale for you, here's the short version.

When I arrived at the University of Colorado, I had never run high mileage. Coach Mark Wetmore knew I had run very low mileage in high school, so he babied me, giving me just 45 to 50 miles a week initially. I did not baby myself, however. Used to running at the front of the pack in high school, I tried to run with Shayne Wille (now Shayne Culpepper), Kelly Smith, and the other far more advanced runners who surrounded me in Boulder. Every workout was like a race for me. I had to redline to keep up, and I refused to fall behind.

My hard work began to pay dividends. At the Big 12 Conference championship meet held in Ames, Iowa, I was our team's third scorer. My mom and several friends from home came to watch the race, and I was so proud of how I performed for them. I was ready to really compete at the college level!

Or not. My hard work quickly began to take its toll. My right shin throbbed on the flight home from Iowa. A couple of weeks later, a stress fracture was diagnosed. By this time, the NCAA championship meet was upon us. Mark assured me that I had earned the right to represent the team in that race and told me that I still could if I wanted to. He knew I was not healthy enough to help the team, but he felt the experience would be valuable for me. So I went ahead and ran and got to experience being beaten by all but 20 of the 180 women in the race. I stopped running for a few weeks to let my leg heal.

By the time I was running again, the indoor track season had begun. I ran a couple of unspectacular races, but my leg started hurting again, so Mark pulled the plug on my season. In the spring it was déjà vu. I got enough healthy training done to run a pretty decent 3,000-meter race at the Mt. San Antonio College (or Mt. Sac) Relays, a major meet for high school, college, and elite athletes held in Southern California in April. My time was only about 10 seconds off the NCAA nationals qualifying standard. "If I can just stay healthy," I told myself, "I could qualify for the national championship meet!"

That turned out to be a big *if*. The pain in my leg returned. I tried to hide it from myself, but I couldn't hide it from others. At a later meet, I bumped into a friend who ran for another college. His eyes quickly dropped from my face to my leg, and he said, "Kara, you're limping! What's wrong?"

"I'm not limping!" I protested. My friend gave me a wary look, as though I might be both injured and crazy.

So my first outdoor track season at Colorado ended early, too. For the next two years, every time I got rolling again on the training and racing front, something big would hit and I felt like I had to start all over again. In my sophomore year, it was anterior compartment syndrome in both legs, which required surgery. In my junior year, it was a severe and long-lasting bout of anemia. It was a pretty awful time for me, punctuated by occasional carefree periods where I actually managed to run pretty well.

At times during those first three years in Boulder, I felt like the most broken-down runner in the world. But, in fact, injuries such as shin splints, muscle strains, and runner's knee are problems that almost all runners experience. Nobody knows exactly how common running injuries are, but I can't think of a single runner I've known who has never been injured.

The reason is that running is a high-impact activity. When you run, you land with a force equal to three to five times your full body weight on each foot eighty to ninety times a minute. That kind of pounding has a way of making your bones, muscles, and joints break down. Some runners are naturally more susceptible to injury, but even the most susceptible runner (take my word for it) can reduce her injury risk and minimize the physical and psychological effects of injuries by managing injury risk and individual injuries properly.

That word *managing* is important. If I have learned only one thing about dealing with injuries, it is that you cannot completely control them. If you expect to prevent all injuries from ever happening, or even just to figure them out instantaneously and overcome them in a day or two, you're only setting yourself up for needless frustration. You're better off having a realistic expectation to manage injuries by doing what you can to prevent the most avoidable ones and having a sensible strategy for dealing with the ones you can't avoid.

The best analogy I can think of is the way firefighters manage wildfires in Colorado and elsewhere. They don't fool themselves into believing that they can completely prevent all wildfires from ever happening. Attempting to do that would require tremendous resources and it still wouldn't work. Instead, the firefighting professionals reduce the risk of wildfires in efficient ways, such as thinning forests and educating the public about fire prevention. And when a fire does break out, firefighters don't try to smother it in one shot, because it's impossible. Instead, they contain the fire and let it burn itself out.

That's how wildfires are managed (I'm told), and you can manage injuries in similar ways—by reducing general risk and "containing" them when they do happen.

# TIPS, TRICKS, AND STRATEGIES TO KEEP YOU INJURY-FREE FOR LIFE

Sometimes I think a lot of nonrunners have this idea that we runners are always injured—or soon will be. That we're constantly twisting our ankles or nursing arthritic knees or rubbing our throbbing shins. Unfortunately, this thinking keeps a lot of people from becoming runners. But it's so not true!

If you're smart about your body and pay attention to the niggling problems before they become big problems, you'll spend very little (if any) time injured. And really, that's a small price to pay for all the wonderful ways running takes care of us—from weight control and stress reduction to bone health and disease prevention. What's an occasional sore calf when weighed against those amazing benefits?

As the preceding pages described, I myself have not been so lucky with injuries. For the first few years after college, I was a mess. You, however—unless you are very, *very* unlucky—will have it way better than me on the injury front.

Read through the following tips and injury prevention strategies, *incorporate* them into your routine, and I guarantee you will stay largely injury-free for a lifetime.

**BE CAREFUL WITH YOUR KNEES:** The best way to protect them is to do exercises to strengthen your quads. Squats are good; squats on a downward-sloping board or hill are even better, as they isolate the inner part of the quadriceps, which is notoriously weak, and a weak quad allows your knee to get out of alignment. Inevitable result: pain, inflammation, time off from running.

**STOP RUNNING FOR AT LEAST TWO DAYS IF YOU FEEL PERSISTENT PAIN AFTER RUNNING:** Soreness or any pain during running doesn't always signal injury, though be aware that it sometimes does. What is more telling is pain after you have finished, especially if it's still there—on the shin, in the knee, or on the top of the foot, for instance—the next day. When this happens, don't run for two full days to see if there's improvement. If so, start back in with a significantly shorter, slower run than normal. You'll likely be fine. If the pain is still there, take two more days off. If the pain is still there after those four days, take a break until the pain is completely gone, however long that takes.

**SOAK IN ICE-COLD WATER ONCE A WEEK:** Coach Salazar is very big on this as a way to control the inflammation and soreness that inevitably occurs with running, especially when you're training hard. I soak in a deep whirlpool-type tube, but putting cold water in the bathtub works just as well. If you can't do it every week, I definitely recommend this after runs over 10 miles to really help you recover quicker.

## IT WORKS FOR ME

I like to aqua jog for 15 to 30 minutes after a long run or a hard track session. I really feel like it helps my muscles recover. I've been known to get in the water and just float around and play. The water pressure feels great on my tired legs and aids recovery.

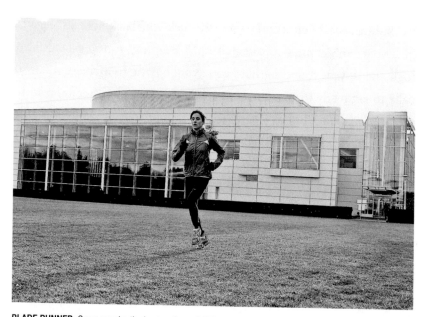

**BLADE RUNNER:** Grass may be the best surface of all for running, as long as it's even and closely mown. Here I work out on the Nike campus.

**RUN ON SOFTER SURFACES SUCH AS DIRT TRAILS RATHER THAN ASPHALT WHEN-EVER POSSIBLE:** This will reduce the pounding your legs are subjected to during training. And some trails are better than others. The trails I ran on in Boulder were mostly hard-packed dirt, and I think they beat my legs up more than the looser dirt trails I now run on in Portland. Grass is probably the best running surface, if it's even (no holes or divots) and closely mowed.

**STRETCH AND STRENGTH TRAIN REGULARLY TO KEEP YOUR BODY IN BALANCE:** This can reduce your injury risk. It's often imbalances such as tight calves and weak hip muscles that make you more susceptible to injuries. I do much more stretching and strength training under Alberto Salazar than I did previously, and it has made my body more resilient.

**TAKE THE GRADUAL APPROACH:** Make a plan with step-by-step increases from week to week. Don't increase your training load every single week, however. Every third or fourth week, cut back your mileage to give your body a chance to catch up. I keep my training load fairly high almost year-round so that I can avoid having to increase it drastically to get ready for races, and even then I set aside three months to prepare for a marathon.

## DEAR KARA

**Right when I start training really well and am starting to get fit, I get injured. It's driving me crazy because I think I could run some good times if I could ever just stay healthy more than three months at a time. What's going on?**

Are they the same injury over and over again or are they different? If they are the same, then you have some weaknesses that you need to address so that you don't continue to fall into this pattern. If they are different, take a look at your training. Each month of training, do you keep pushing it harder and harder? Make sure you aren't pushing things too far and that you are getting plenty of recovery. It might be that you get through two months, start to get excited, and then start pushing too hard. If you don't keep a training log, start doing so. Then you can look for patterns to see if there are mistakes you are making. Take the time for the supplemental things like strength drills and stretching. Good luck!

**LISTEN TO YOUR BODY:** A smart training plan is no guarantee against aches and pains. These will sometimes pop up when you least expect them. And when they do pop up, you need to be ready and willing to obey the message they are trying to send you: "Something's wrong!" and change your training so that those aches and pains don't become full-blown injuries. The most common overuse injuries don't happen suddenly; they develop slowly over a period of many days or even weeks. Thus you usually have plenty of warning, but you need to heed that warning.

**LEARN TO DISTINGUISH GARDEN-VARIETY SORENESS FROM THE PAIN THAT SIGNIFIES AN INJURY:** This obviously relates to the previous tip about listening to your body. The key is to become a *discerning* listener, as not every ache and pain requires time off. A certain amount of soreness is a normal part of training and is usually nothing to worry about. And while it is crucial to take time off when needed, you don't want to miss runs because of overreacting.

**ASK QUESTIONS AND GET HELP:** And keep pushing for answers if things aren't getting better. Running injuries are often hard to diagnose. For example, there are lots of different injuries that can make your knee hurt. I had compartment syndrome for a year before it was correctly diagnosed. Read up on your symptoms and on the various injuries that match them. Pay attention to every detail of your injury, and share those details with your doctors. You never know which small clue will unravel the mystery of what's wrong. The more time and effort you put into solving the mystery of a current injury, the faster you will get it fixed and the sooner you will be running again.

## DEAR KARA

**Is there an injury or injuries that women get more than men that I should watch out for? If so, how can I protect myself from it?**
In the group that I train in, the men and women get injured the same amount and have the same injuries. One thing I'd recommend to women is to take an iron supplement. Because of our menstrual cycles, we lose more blood and are at a higher risk of anemia.

**CONSIDER DROPPING DOWN TO THREE OR FOUR DAYS A WEEK OF RUNNING IF YOU KEEP GETTING INJURED AT FIVE TO SEVEN DAYS A WEEK:** Point being here, as mentioned before, that you need to make adjustments if something isn't working, like running every day. It's commendable that you are committed to doing this, but if you keep getting injured at that frequency, change the frequency! The great news is, if you add vigorous cross-training such as swimming or cycling, you'll gain better all-around fitness and should decrease your injury risk.

## DEAR KARA

**I think that running has become too much a part of my self-image. It's fine now, because I can run, but what if one day I can't run anymore because of injury. What will I do?**

Always remember that running is something that you do and love, but not what defines you. I learned this lesson early on. In high school I went from "the runner" to not knowing who I was because I couldn't run due to an injury. Now I say I am a person who loves to run. It is one of many things that make me who I am, but it does not define me. Get in touch with your other interests and hobbies. It might be music, cooking, friendship, and so on. The possibilities are endless. Just remember that you are so much more than a person who likes to run.

**KEEP TRAINING WHEN YOU CAN'T RUN:** Okay, I hate cross-training, but it still beats sitting around, getting depressed, and falling out of shape when I'm injured, so I do it. You might consider it also. Ironically, it's my love of running that motivates me to swim, aqua jog, and use the elliptical trainer, because cross-training helps me return to running fitter and faster. While simulating running in a most unsatisfying way on the elliptical trainer or in the pool, I remind myself over and over,

"This is for your running. This is for your running." Try it—or any other trick that works for you.

**MIX IT UP WHILE YOU'RE AT IT:** This is so key! The more variety you can incorporate into your cross-training, the less unpleasant it will be. There are those who say that injured runners should choose cross-training activities that are similar to running, such as elliptical training, because the fitness benefit you get from them will transfer back to running. That's good advice, but I don't think you will get as much benefit from elliptical training or whatever else if you're bored to death doing it, so I recommend that you do whatever you enjoy most, or better yet, do a mix of different activities to stave off boredom. Consider switching them every 5 to 10 minutes during your session.

**LEARN WHERE YOUR *CUTOFF* IS AND DON'T GO BEYOND IT:** By *cutoff* I mean that level of training (usually it's a weekly mileage level) where you know you're at real risk of injury if you go past it. It's always possible to raise that cutoff point by learning what parts of your body need to be strengthened—and then doing that—but unless you're very diligent about this, the more important step is to stay below the problem threshold in the first place.

**STAY POSITIVE AND NEVER GIVE UP:** When I was younger, I used to focus on the races and workouts I was missing, the fitness draining out of me day after day, the loss of camaraderie with my teammates. Basically that attitude didn't get me anywhere except depressed. Now I think about what I can do to heal faster and to stay fit while I am healing. I work on creating a plan to get back into racing shape after I return to normal training. This doesn't wipe away all of the frustration of being injured, but it sure helps.

# DEAR KARA

**A guy in my training group said recently that women get injured more than men because they're weaker and have worse biomechanics. Is this true?**

If we are so weak, then why would God have chosen us to carry babies? One thing women do have that men don't is our hips, which can cause some rotation when we are running, and if this is excessive, it can lead to injuries. But it's no different than a man who overpronates. Tell the guy in your group that he's wrong on this one!

**STAY CONNECTED TO RUNNING:** To minimize the isolation you may feel when you can't run, keep in touch with your training partners. Call them on the days when you normally would have run with them. Or go to your running club meetings just to keep up with the gossip. Go to races and cheer for your friends. It might seem like this would be torture, but you might be surprised how good it feels to be part of the support crew for a change.

**OR GET AWAY FROM IT FOR A WHILE!** That's right—sometimes it's better to go in the opposite direction. When recovering from longer injuries especially, really getting away from running may feel better than trying to stay involved with it. I learned this lesson in 2001. Adam and I were recently married and I was struggling through yet another long injury bout. I reached a point where even thinking about running hurt, so I decided to cultivate other parts of my life. Figuring that being married was a good excuse to learn to cook, I learned to cook. Instead of making myself miserable with pathetic wishes that my body would heal faster than it realistically could, I dedicated myself to becoming a more well-rounded person. Fortunately, running is not our entire lives. Not being able to run temporarily because of injury offers opportunities. Be determined to make the most of them.

**HAVE FAITH IN YOUR BODY:** One simple reminder helps me stay sane when I'm injured. *My body knows how to heal itself.* Runners can get a little irrational at times—you know, like when we're injured! We start to think that what is broken in us will never be fixed. "Just my luck: I've got the first case of runner's knee that will never heal!" But "career-ending" injuries in runners are extremely rare. Hang in there. Trust your body. It may need time, but it knows what it's doing.

## ON THE CONTRARY

**Sometimes your coach doesn't know best.** There are days where your body just says no, or you have something that is sore and you know you shouldn't train through it. You should always listen to your body over your coach.

**Instead of just jumping into an ice bath right after a hard session, I think it's better to get in the pool or do some stretches first.** If you go straight to the ice, you are just going to tighten yourself up. Move around and stretch out first.

**EASE BACK INTO TRAINING:** This is key, because we're never more likely to get injured than when returning to running after an injury. Cruel, I know. First of all, there is the chance of reinjuring the part of your body that just healed. Tissue damage can linger long after pain disappears. Then there's the greater risk of developing new and different injuries. Even a couple of weeks without running can make your bones, muscles, and joints a little less tolerant of the stress of repetitive impact. Trying to pick up right where you left off in your training is usually a big mistake, because your legs are no longer the same. They need a chance to gently reacquaint themselves with the stress of running. So come back *slowly*.

107

REMEMBER THE HARD–EASY RULE, BUT MAKE IT HARD–EASY–EASY: One of the oldest and smartest adages in running is always take a really easy day after you run either long or hard. The idea is that this allows your body and mind a chance to recover and rebuild so that they come back stronger than ever. But really it's a good idea to follow a hard day with at least *two* easy days, one of which might involve no running at all. This will ensure you're completely rested and ready for the next challenging run. If it's important to you to burn some extra calories every day, just do some cross-training that requires minimal or no pounding on your legs. Examples: walking, swimming, strength training, stationary cycling, elliptical training, or regular cycling.

## DEAR KARA

**I'm concerned that running is eventually going to give me varicose veins. Does this happen? If so, would it help to wear those compression socks like Paula Radcliffe used to wear?**

I'm no doctor, but I don't think that running is going to give you varicose veins. If running does cause your legs to swell, then compression socks might be something to consider. My legs and ankles started to swell in my eighth month of pregnancy, so I did start wearing compression socks for the rest of my pregnancy.

GIVE YOURSELF A LIFT: If you tend to get Achilles tendon tenderness on occasion, you may do well to put a quarter-inch firm pad under the heel area of your running shoes. (Place the pad underneath the removable sock liner of the shoe so that it doesn't move around.) Raising up your heel will allow the Achilles to shorten slightly, which will take a little stress off it during each running stride. A heel pad can also help with tenderness in and around the heel itself, which is sometimes associated with plantar fasciitis (see page 120). Always put heel pads in

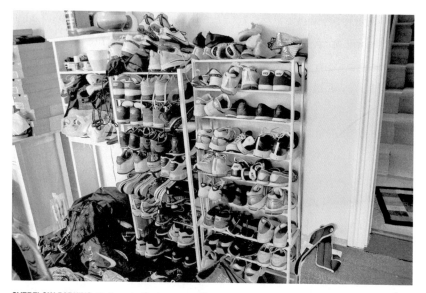

**OVERFLOW PARKING:** It's important to leave your shoes on the rack and regularly walk barefoot to keep your feet and lower legs strong. Here, our tools of the trade.

both shoes—even if you're only having problems on one side—so as not to create a leg-length imbalance.

**WALK IN BARE FEET REGULARLY:** Think about it: your feet spend a large majority of their "walking" time trapped in shoes that end up doing a lot of their work for them. Running shoes themselves are often touted as providing maximum support and cushioning, and so on. Thus it's no surprise that there's a growing movement in the running community to run barefoot. And not just on grass as part of your cooldown but all the time. The idea is that we were meant to run barefoot—after all, we did it for thousands of years before dual-density midsole and cantilevered footbridge came along to rescue us. But regardless of whether you plan to go all the way with this, it's smart to give your feet a regular workout by walking barefoot for part of each day. This will strengthen your feet and lower legs and help bolster them against injury.

**BE KIND TO YOUR FEET IN OTHER WAYS AS WELL:** Your feet are truly "where the rubber hits the road" in running—your point of contact as it were. With most runners averaging about 1,500 steps per mile of running, that's a lot of pounding on your feet, so take care of your togs with the occasional foot soak in ice-cold water (helps with any inflammation) or in a warm salt bath. A weekly foot massage and regular pedicure do wonders also.

**BE OKAY WITH REGULAR BREAKS FROM RUNNING:** Running isn't going any-where, so don't stress if you have to miss a few days or even a week. You won't lose any fitness in that amount of time, and sometimes the break is just what the doctor ordered. Have an overseas business trip coming up and you're worried about fitting in your running? Maybe hit the hotel gym for some treadmill time, but if that doesn't work out, don't sweat it. Anticipating a busy week with family visiting and not sure when you'll be able to run? Take those days off! Again, running will be there for you. Have faith that you'll get back to it soon enough. Meanwhile, a break could be just the thing.

# DEAR KARA

**I don't get injured often and I want to keep it that way. What are the three best strength exercises I can do to keep me from getting injured? Or is there something else you do besides strength work that is more effective for injury prevention?**

Good question! We all have different weaknesses, but if I had to pick my top three exercises to stay healthy, they would be calf raises, body squats, and lunges. They really work the lower body and keep things strong. My other recommendation would be to take the time to stretch after you run. This is essential for helping to keep the body flexible and injury-free. Good luck!

**GO EASY ON THE STRETCHING:** Research has shown that you can actually increase your injury risk if you stretch too aggressively. We've all seen those runners who look like they're trying to get in a workout and hit their target heart rate during a stretching routine. Not good. Whatever your preferred method of stretching (static, active-isolated, etc.), go at it slowly and deliberately.

**DO IT JUST BEFORE GOING TO BED:** One problem runners often have with stretching is when to fit it in. For me it works best to do a stretching session just before I hit the sack at night. It relaxes me, and I find that I wake up in the morning feeling less stiff if I have stretched the night before. Stretching helps prevent injuries caused by tightness in the muscles and tendons and also guards against the loss of range of motion that comes with aging.

## DEAR KARA

I'm an older runner (age sixty-seven) and I'm worried that running is going to cause osteoporosis and stress fractures. Is this crazy? I just started running three years ago and love it so much. I don't want to give it up.

I'm no doctor, but I think that if you have been running for three years without any problems, I don't know why you would have problems now. Just be sure you are getting plenty of calcium in your diet. You go, girl!

## HERE'S THE RUB: A MASSAGE PRIMER

*Al Kupczak is the massage therapist for the Nike Oregon Project team of elite distance runners. He's been working with me off and on (but mostly on) since I was a junior at the University of Colorado. Here is Kupczak's advice on massage:*

**FIND A GOOD THERAPIST:** Word of mouth is your best bet. Ask other runners who they see. Get details about how the therapist works, how easy it is to get an appointment, and how long he or she has been in business. Or you can find a therapist near you by going to the American Massage Therapy Association at amtamassage.org and using their "Find a Massage Therapist" tool.

**WEAR WHAT YOU'RE COMFORTABLE WITH:** Most of the time, runners will wear running shorts and maybe a top. But some runners don't wear anything, and the therapist will use a towel to cover areas he or she is working on.

**STAY IN CONTROL:** You're the client, and you have the power. If a therapist tries to tell you what to do or wants to make you do something you're not comfortable with, that's wrong.

**"LISTEN" TO THEIR HANDS:** You should feel confidence in the therapist's hands. If he or she doesn't feel comfortable, you'll be able to tell. Likewise, if you're not comfortable, a good massage therapist will know. If any of this is going on, it can be a long hour, so be sure to mention it right away if anything is bothering you.

**EXPECT IT TO FEEL GOOD:** Sometimes there will be discomfort, but this should be the exception. The idea that you're going into a "torture chamber" and aren't getting a proper massage unless you're yelling and screaming is just not true. Still, some runners are into that, like it's a macho thing. And some massage therapists will cater to that, because that's what the runner wants. I think that's silly.

**GO WITH THE FLOW:** Says Kupczak: "It has happened countless times where I'll be running my hand along a runner's calf, for instance, and she'll yell, 'There! That's it! That's where it hurts! Do you feel that?' And yes, I'll usually feel it, but it's not always easy to describe what it is exactly. With experience, therapists learn how these things feel and we know what to do about them, but it's tough to put these things into words. Sometimes I'll describe the problem area and what I'm doing for it just to give the person something to hang on to, but the subtleties of massage therapy don't always lend themselves to words."

## DEAR KARA

**I have enough money in my monthly budget to either get a massage or see a chiropractor once a week, and I really feel like I need both given my injury history. In the past, both kept me healthy! So which should I choose? Or do you think there's another specialist that might be better?**

This is a tough question. You might want to consider an active release techniques (ART) therapist, which is a combination of both. But there are also massage therapists who can do some adjustments. If you really feel like they are both helping you out, trade each month. And ask your massage therapist and your chiropractor for stretches or exercises you can be doing to bridge the gap between sessions.

## WHAT MASSAGE WILL DO FOR YOU

*If you always thought massage felt good but didn't do a lot for your running, you may've been going to the wrong person. My longtime massage therapist, Al Kupczak, explains the benefits.*

- **You'll recover faster.** A weekly massage will help you recover from your workouts faster and more completely. That's because massage increases blood flow, which in turn gets more oxygen to your muscles, which revives them. This is also why massage can help you recover from injuries faster.

- **You'll feel good.** You knew this one already! Running can be a tough thing to do, and not just for elite-level runners like Kara. It's unforgiving at times, especially if you're putting in a lot of miles or ramping up for a marathon. So for a lot of people, their weekly massage is a treat. It's something they look forward to. It makes them

113

feel good. And if it helps them with their recovery and their training, so much the better, from their point of view.

- **You'll lower your injury risk.** Skeptics don't believe this, but it is absolutely true. I can't tell you how many times I have noticed little aches and pains in runners, and I can take care of them before they become full-blown injuries. Most common running injuries don't happen suddenly. They take time to develop, but you may not notice them in the early stages. A good massage therapist notices them and can do something about them.

- **You'll get valuable feedback.** There will be times when you're feeling pain and the massage therapist can't help you. But what he or she can do is refer you to the right specialist. I actually like when this happens because it gets me off the hook. Sometimes it's good to remind runners—and myself—that I can't cure everything. And I definitely can't, but I can help you find someone who can. I most frequently refer runners to osteopaths (they understand the whole body) and chiropractors (when things are seriously out of alignment, there's only so much I can do).

- **You'll run better.** Ah, the benefit you've been waiting for. But keep your head on this one. A lot of really good runners think massage therapists are the final piece of the puzzle that is going to send them right to the top. Unfortunately, some massage therapists will lead runners on that this is the case. Not true. But we can help a little bit. We can help you get faster. How?

By increasing your range of motion and thus your running efficiency

By increasing your blood flow so that more oxygen reaches your running muscles

By making your connective tissue (tendons and ligaments) more supple and responsive

## IS ART THERAPY FOR YOU?

*I swear by it and receive regular ART from my therapist, Justin Whittaker. ART has helped me out of some very tough injury jams, and I'm convinced it's been key to my health the last few years, despite very intense training. Here's the low-down from Whittaker.*

ART stands for active release techniques. This relatively new, hands-on treatment similar to massage is used to treat injuries to the soft tissues of the body, including the muscles, ligaments, fascia, and nerves. Practitioners believe ART is especially suited to runners because it helps locate and treat scar tissue adhesions that accumulate in the muscles and surrounding soft tissue. Once the problem area is located, the goal of ART is to:

- break up restrictive adhesions
- reinstate normal tissue flexibility and movement
- restore flexibility, balance, and stability to the injured area and to the entire kinetic chain

Some describe ART as "active massage," because the person getting treatment moves during the session. The practitioner will first shorten the muscle, tendon, or ligament, and then apply a very specific pressure with his or her hands as you stretch and lengthen the tissues. As the tissue lengthens, the practitioner assesses the texture and tension of the muscle to determine if the tissue is healthy or contains scar tissue that requires further treatment. The practitioner then can treat abnormal tissues by combining precisely directed tension with specific patient movements.

ART also allows the practitioner to assess and correct problems in other areas of the kinetic chain that may be contributing to the original problem. In this way, the practitioner can address all the soft tissues that have become dysfunctional and are contributing to the original injury, even if those other areas are not yet causing pain.

I believe ART works well for runners, especially when you combine it with supplemental stretching and strengthening exercises. Although each case is different, and different injuries heal at different rates, we usually see significant improvements in just four to six treatments, which is why so many elite athletes and professional sports teams now have ART practitioners on staff.

115

# ART Comes to the Rescue

*With a painful injury threatening to derail my Olympic Trials hopes, I turned to a relatively new therapy for help.*

**The context:** It's the 2008 Olympic Trials at legendary Hayward Field in Eugene, Oregon. On the evening of July 2, I'm stricken with severe hip pain that emanates down the outside of my left leg. I'd finished second in the 10,000 a week before to qualify for the Olympic team, but desperately wanted to compete in the 5,000 in two days' time, in hopes of avenging my loss to rival Shalane Flanagan in the earlier race.

Along with the pain, I have severe range-of-motion issues. I remember trying to do some strides that evening of the second, and my knee totally locked up. I just stopped running, put my sweats on, and called Justin in a panic.

Portland-based chiropractor Justin Whittaker is my ART therapist. He'd been seeing me for several years at that point, and has been helping to keep me healthy since. Here's how those anxious moments at the Trials played out, as remembered by Whittaker:

## July 2

When I reach Kara at the track, she is complaining of left hip soreness with additional pain down the iliotibial band (ITB) to the knee. The problem has been intermittent for two weeks due to the intense training buildup in preparation for the Trials. Kara is now right on the edge of keeping things as functional as possible. There is no time for normal therapy and recovery. The hip had held up pretty well but was regressing quickly, thanks to the hard 10,000-meter race effort the week before, followed by the qualifying round of the 5,000 meters earlier tonight.

## The Diagnosis

Here's what I find out when I examine her. The problem stems from her gluteus me-dius and tensor fascia lata (TFL) muscles, which rest against each other on the front of the hip. They both help to flex and control the hip, but their respective movements can create tension where they overlap. This tension can alter the function of both muscles and cause small adhesions to form. With continued stress, the problem can spread to the surrounding muscles, which is what has happened to Kara, re-sulting in altered mechanics down to her left knee. I'm worried that her knee could sustain damage from the stress.

## The Treatment

She had massage treatment earlier in the evening, which has helped, but the knee pain is not coming under control. It is now 11:30 P.M. My plan is to treat the areas of her hip, ITB, and knee to normalize the movement patterns between the muscles and try to restore full range of motion (ROM). When I check her hip ROM, it is reduced by 50 percent in rotation. It's clear that the joint is now locked down by the surrounding muscle. I perform ART to help separate the tissues, clear the ITB tension, and mobilize the hip and knee joints. This is not an easy procedure for Kara. She's in a lot of pain.

## July 3

### The Treatment Continues

In the evening we revisit the injury area and find that it is improving. The question looms whether she will be ready for her race the next day. After further treatment with ART, we agree to meet before her race the following day to see where things stand.

## July 4

### The Treatment Continues

It is race day. The leg has progressed well. We work through the same series of muscles of the past two sessions. Her ROM is better and the muscle function is improving. Because we are so close to her race, I have to decrease the intensity of ART therapy. I have done my best in a short time frame. The real test will be in the final laps of the race when fatigue sets in. I'm especially worried about the final 100 meters, when Kara will accelerate to near top speed.

## The Race

After a tense, closely contested race, Kara closes hard and wins by two strides. The happy ending flashes on the Jumbo screen at the south end of Hayward Field. Kara has emphatically punched her ticket to Beijing with a 5,000-meter win in 15:01.02. It's July 4. The celebration begins.

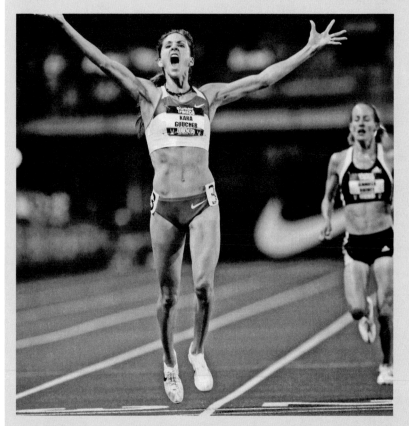

**A YELLING MOMENT:** Thanks in large part to (literally) 11th-hour ART therapy, I battled through a painful injury to win the 2008 Olympic Trials 5,000 meters.

# Overcoming the Most Common Running Injuries

Of course, it's best to bypass these altogether if you can (you'll find smart strategies for doing that elsewhere in this chapter), but if you do get injured, don't sweat it! Chances are you'll be back on the road in no time—if you're diligent about your rehab. For each of these injuries, you simply need to (1) stop running (and perhaps cross-train) until the pain goes away, then (2) start back to running gradually, and (3) follow the simple-but-effective treatment plan below.

## Achilles Tendinitis

### What You Feel

Persistent pain in the back of the ankle, usually near the heel.

### Treatment Plan

- Ice at least twice a day for 15 to 20 minutes each time.
- Take anti-inflammatories (aspirin, ibuprofen, naproxen sodium, etc.) as directed on the label.
- Place a quarter-inch heel pad in the shoe of the affected leg; this will take some of the stress off the Achilles tendon, as it won't have to stretch quite as much during every running stride.
- Gently stretch the calf and Achilles tendon using the classic runner's against-the-wall stretch on page 52.
- Once you're completely in the clear, strengthen the calf and Achilles with calf raises on a weight machine or off the edge of a step.

119

## Iliotibial Band Syndrome

### What You Feel

Pain on the outside of the knee.

## Treatment Plan

- Ice at least twice a day for 15 to 20 minutes each time (unlike some other injuries, ITB syndrome usually responds quite well to icing).
- Take anti-inflammatories (aspirin, ibuprofen, naproxen sodium, etc.) as directed on the label.
- Stretch the ITB by lying on your back and placing the foot of the affected leg on top of the opposite knee, then reaching down and "pulling" the knee of the affected leg up toward your face. Hold the stretch for 2 to 3 seconds, then release. Repeat 10 times.
- Strengthen the gluteus medius muscle near the hip by lying on your side and lifting the upper leg straight up from the floor, scissor style. Hold for 10 seconds, then release. Repeat 10 times.

# Plantar Fasciitis

## What You Feel

Sharp pain in the arch area, usually back near the heel

## Treatment Plan

- Ice at least twice a day for 15 to 20 minutes each time (preferably once right after running).
- Take anti-inflammatories (aspirin, ibuprofen, naproxen sodium, etc.) as directed on the label.
- Stretch the calf using the runner's against-the-wall stretch on page 52 (*note:* tight calf muscles are often a contributing factor to plantar fasciitis).
- Stretch and massage the arch area by rolling your foot firmly over a golf ball for 5 minutes twice a day.
- Trying using a sleep sock that keeps your foot flexed during the night.
- *Cautionary note:* Plantar fasciitis may be the toughest of these five injuries to overcome, so carefully follow your treatment plan. You *will* see progress, but you need to be diligent with your rehab.

# Runner's Knee (sometimes called chondromalacia)

## What You Feel

Pain around or just beneath the kneecap, especially after sitting bent-legged for a long time or when walking downstairs.

## Treatment Plan

- Ice at least twice a day for 15 to 20 minutes each time.
- Take anti-inflammatories (aspirin, ibuprofen, naproxen sodium, etc.) as directed on the label.
- Try to avoid downhill running until you're completely healed.
- Stretch the quadriceps muscle just above the knee using the ankle grab stretch on page 53.
- Strengthen the quadriceps to help stabilize the kneecap. Half-squats on a downhill slope or a decline board (i.e., facing downhill) may be the best quad strengthener.

# Shin Splints

## What You Feel

Persistent pain along one or both shins (*note:* this injury is very common among beginning runners).

## Treatment Plan

- Ice at least twice a day for 15 to 20 minutes each time (as with ITB syndrome, shin splints normally respond very well to ice).
- Take anti-inflammatories (aspirin, ibuprofen, naproxen sodium, etc.) as directed on the label.
- Stretch the shin muscles by flexing (pointing) your foot down and away from you as far as you can flex it, holding for 3 seconds, then releasing. Repeat 10 times. Then point your foot up and back toward your body as far as you can, hold for 3 seconds, then release. Repeat 10 times.
- Strengthen the shin muscles using my alphabet exercise on page 12 and by alternating walking on your toes and walking on your heels for 20 seconds each time.

# Kupczak on Kara

*Massage therapist Al Kupczak works with several team members of the Nike Oregon Project, including me. Here's his take on the 2:25 marathoner:*

- Coach Salazar pushes Kara hard. So when she's in her peak training season, I'll see her twice a week, sometimes three, when we include a stretching session.
- As with a lot of distance runners, I'm very careful about her high hamstring area. When this gets tight, she can't extend her legs as freely with each stride.
- Kara is very particular about her training. Very meticulous. She is always willing to take the extra step, to do all the little things you need to do to get better.
- With a lot of runners, they care about the running and that's it. Kara cares about everything she does.
- I can't ever see Kara doing anything illegal to make herself faster because she's too tough for that. She likes to prove herself, and she would see performance-enhancing drugs as taking the shortcut. She never takes the shortcut. She does what needs to be done—and then some.

# CHAPTER 5

# BALANCING RUNNING AND LIFE

I am not a runner. I am a person who runs. Running is an important part of my self, but only one part. This perspective is not incompatible with my desire to be the best runner I can possibly be. Make no mistake: I don't want to look back at my career in twenty years and realize that I could have been better and achieved more. I am determined to realize 100 percent of my running potential. But I think that I would run worse, not better, if I allowed running to completely dominate my life.

Athletes are not machines. We are people. And like all people, we need much more than to achieve goals in sports. If we put too much of ourselves into training and competition, those other needs are not met. When important needs go unmet, we become unhappy, and when we're unhappy, we do not perform well as athletes. See how that works?

Mark Wetmore understands the importance of nourishing the whole person. A well-rounded person himself, he always used to stress the importance of having diverse interests with his runners. He frequently recommended books to us and took a genuine interest in the things we learned in our classes. He was preaching to the choir with me. I always enjoyed school and I absolutely loved reading. I made the smart choice to major in the subject that most interested me—psychology—instead of majoring in whatever subject I felt would be most practical in terms of preparing me for a future career.

Because I enjoyed psychology, I gladly worked hard in my classes and earned a 4.0 grade-point average in my final year. In that year I took a class that covered Alberto Bandura's theory of self-efficacy. This is the idea that people tend to have pretty accurate notions about how well they can perform specific tasks, because we learn our capabilities from doing those tasks and because these notions are self-fulfilling. For example, you probably won't win a race you don't think you can win, even if you really could. As you might imagine, I was excited about the relevance of this idea to the mental side of my running, and I applied it with some success.

That is one specific example of how maintaining a rich life outside of running can help a person's running. But even when reading and other intellectual interests do not provide such obvious tools, they help by creating a happier, more balanced person.

Many great runners do a lot more than run. The men's marathon world record holder, Haile Gebrselassie, has a huge business empire in Ethiopia. One of the top American runners of the 1990s, Bob Kempainen, juggled training and racing with medical school. I am no business mogul or doctor, but until I graduated from CU, I was not completely settled on focusing exclusively on running afterward. I applied for and was offered a postgraduate scholarship in psychology, and turning it down to focus on my running was a tough decision. I still read *Psychology Today*, though, and a whole lot more. I received a Kindle for my last birthday and it's been practically glued to my face ever since!

Another passion of mine is food—yes, I'm a foodie—and wine. I love to cook. My massage therapist went to cooking school and is always giving me new recipes to try. I could easily go to IKEA every

Saturday and come home with a backseat full of kitchen toys. Adam and I took some classes on wine appreciation together. We don't drink a lot, but we really enjoy the little we do drink, as well as the whole process of exploring wines.

My cooking has some practical carryover to my running, too. Nutrition is a crucial piece of the performance puzzle. You can't run your best with a bad diet. Knowing how to cook and preparing most of the food I eat enables me to control my diet and ensure that it supports my running. But I would cook regardless, because I enjoy it. Again, though, I believe that merely enjoying things outside of running helps my running by keeping me balanced and fulfilled as a complete person.

Some runners look at their running as competing against the other parts of their life. I try not to. I try to live my life as a unity of parts, where every part contributes to the whole. The purpose of my life is to be happy, to be the best overall person I can be, and to contribute something positive to the world. Running is one component of my life that helps me realize my purpose. But the other parts do, too: my marriage, my other important relationships, my work with kids, my reading, my cooking, and all the rest. Everything fits together. I know that my relationship with Adam helps my running and that my running helps my relationship with Adam, that my youth mentoring helps my running and vice versa, and so forth. Sometimes I do find that one part of my life starts to take away from the others. Then I try to restore the right balance as quickly as possible.

There's something in us that knows what's best for us in most situations. Call it the heart. We have lots of different instincts and desires that make choices difficult at times, but I find that if I listen within myself intently enough, I can always discern what my heart really wants, sooner or later. To keep the right balance in my life I follow my heart, and you can, too.

There's no better example than my decision to start a family with Adam. The decision to have a child is an especially difficult one for professional runners, because we have to essentially take a one-year sabbatical from our career, which is short enough to begin with. Getting pregnant is a big deal for any working woman (or any nonworking woman, for that matter), but it poses a special challenge for those who make a living by running races.

Adam and I knew that we wanted to have a child from the very beginning. The only question was when. Most runners who are fortunate enough to make a real career in running prefer to get well established in their career before they call a time-out for pregnancy. Adam and I agreed that I should follow this strategy. The obvious best time would be after the 2004 Olympics in Athens. I would be twenty-six then, and with the Olympics checked off my dream list, I would surely be ready for motherhood. Even with a year off, I would have plenty of time to prepare for the next Olympics.

Except I didn't qualify for the 2004 Games. After that disappointment, I asked myself if I should go ahead and try to get pregnant anyway, but my heart told me loud and clear to *keep running*. I knew Adam was ready and I felt bad about asking him to wait, but we both understood that since I would carry the child, we needed to follow my heart before his.

Happily, I made the 2008 Olympic team, and I ran pretty well in Beijing. But my ninth- and tenth-place finishes in the 5000m and the 10,000m, respectively, left me unsatisfied. By that time, Alberto Salazar and I had decided that the marathon might be my best distance, but I hadn't run one yet. I came home from Beijing with a burning desire to run a marathon. Top-10 wasn't good enough. I wanted to win something big, and my best chance was in the marathon, and the time was now.

I asked Adam to wait just a little longer. As he always does, he supported my wish. I wasn't asking him to wait long. The 2008 ING New York City Marathon took place less than three months after the Olympics. I ran well in New York, but my third-place finish left me even hungrier than I was before. Again, there was no mistaking the message of my heart to *keep running*.

I told Adam, "This time I'm serious. I need just one more race. I learned a lot from New York. I think I can really nail my next marathon." Once more, Adam told me he understood and supported my choice, but I hated making him wait. I felt I was taking fatherhood away from him. Even so, I knew the regret of stopping now would feel even worse.

I ran the Boston Marathon the next spring and lost by nine seconds. Nine seconds! I broke into tears as soon as I crossed the finish line. I cried not only because the fulfillment of a dream had been snatched away from me when I could already taste it. I also cried because I knew what I would have to tell Adam that night.

"I swear, just one more race!" I told him. I felt like a monster. How could I do this to my husband? Perhaps I was kidding myself. There

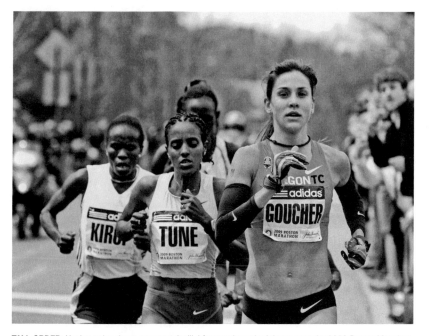

**TALL ORDER:** Hoping to break my opponents' will, I frequently pushed the pace at the 2009 Boston Marathon. I got outkicked at the end, and finished third.

127

**BALANCING RUNNING AND LIFE**

would always be another race to run. Was I too selfish to even be a mother? Why else would I keep putting running ahead of bearing my first child?

In my heart of hearts, though, I knew that what I was doing was right—for me, for Adam, and for the baby to come. It was because motherhood was so important to me that I did not want to enter into it until I was truly ready. I never really lost trust that I would be ready eventually. But I had to follow my heart. It was just taking my heart a little longer than expected to tell me the time had come!

I ran the World Championship Marathon in Berlin four months after Boston. It was a bad day for me and I finished tenth. Instead of taking the last step forward to win my first major marathon, I took two steps backward. As soon as I crossed the finish line, I knew I was ready to be a mom. No regrets.

I hope the tips and strategies in the rest of this chapter will help you achieve balance between your running and the rest of your life.

# BEST WAYS TO STAY IN PERFECT TUNE WITH YOUR RUNNING AND YOUR LIFE

You hear it a lot from women runners that running is their escape, their outlet, their sanity time. Once I heard a woman say that running was the only time in her life when she felt truly herself—happy, calm, and confident.

When I hear these things—and believe me I've had thoughts like these in the past—on the one hand, it makes me appreciate the incredible power that running has, and how important and wonderful it can be in our lives. Who doesn't need sanity time? But on the other hand, I would suggest that if you feel like this a lot—that running is your one escape—you probably need to take a closer look at what you're escaping from. It may be time to make some adjustments and shift priorities to make your life a little easier on you.

What's more, making running your escape hatch to Sanityville puts a big burden on your running! What if you get injured and can't run for a while? What if your running goes a little stale and you need a break from it? What then? What becomes your outlet at that point?

This chapter offers some ways to organize your running and the rest of your life into a coherent, integrated whole. I hope you find them useful.

**KNOW YOUR PRIORITIES:** There are only so many hours in a day, and on a practical level the various parts of our lives do compete with each other for time. If you feel like there's just too much going on and it's hurting your running (among other things), a good place to start is to simply make a list of your priorities. Sometimes just seeing them written down can help you get a handle on them. Then it's time to . . .

**SORT YOUR PRIORITIES:** Some runners I know operate in a constant state of low-grade anxiety because they care about all the parts of their lives—job, children, running, and so on—but they feel like each part is always encroaching on the others. Thus they can't really enjoy their runs because they feel they have to rush through them to spend quality time with their kids. And their family time is marred because they feel guilty about wanting to get away for a short run. This is when it's time to *prioritize* your priorities so that they can more easily coexist with each other. That list of priorities you made? Put them in order from most important to least, then try to live according to that order.

# I LOVE THIS QUOTE

Besides, a medal is only a thing, an object. The race, the achievement, is what's most important. I think the medal is still on the floor of my car, among the diapers.
>    —Joan Nesbit, after skipping the World Indoor 3,000m awards
>    ceremony to return home to her two-year-old daughter, Sarah Jane

I love this quote because I feel the same way. I love the memory of winning the bronze medal at the World Championships in 2007. The memory brings tears to my eyes. But the medal does nothing for me. In fact, a few months ago I was doing an interview at my home and I was asked to get it out to show it. Adam and I searched the house up and down and couldn't find it. I just found it as I was cleaning out my closet to move to a new house. It was under a pile of sweatpants.

**KEEP YOUR RUNNING IN PERSPECTIVE:** This might sound a little strange coming from someone who makes her living from running, but running is not the most important part of my life. Occasionally, however, I think and act like it is, which inevitably puts running in conflict with other parts of my life and creates anxiety. At these moments, I have to step back and tell myself, "Running isn't going to tuck you in at night, Kara." That's my way of remembering that missing a run here or there is not the end of the world. So my advice to you is, being fully conscious of your priorities will help you be at peace with not always being able to do it all.

**CULTIVATE YOUR PASSIONS:** It's so important to have something else that you are equally as passionate about. Most successful people have something; it helps keep your mind and body fresh so that you can enjoy your running. Jack Nicklaus, the famous golfer, has always been addicted to fly fishing. It's not possible to run every minute of every day, so find something (other than work!) that you can use to divert your attention so that you come back to running feeling energized.

**SEEK HAPPINESS:** Happy runners are successful runners. If you want the performance to be as close to perfect as possible, it is essential that your mind is on board, too. Make sure the other areas of your life are as balanced and close to perfect as possible so that you are confident of achieving happiness and contentment.

## ON THE CONTRARY

**You can get too focused on running.** Some people want to get better and get too obsessed with it. I find I run my best and I enjoy my life better when I have other interests.

## DEAR KARA

**I'm training for a marathon and also have a demanding job as an attorney. Unfortunately my busy schedule is having an effect on my sex drive and my husband has definitely noticed. Anything I can do about it? (I want to run this marathon!)**

Life stress, especially physical stress, can have an effect on your sex drive. When I am running 120 miles a week, it can definitely put a damper on mine! One thing I have learned—if your husband starts it, go with it. You may not have the drive to start something, but once you get going, you'll be glad that you did!

**TALK ABOUT OTHER THINGS:** If you only ever talk about running, it won't be long before your friendship circle starts to get smaller and you get less support for your passion. Keep it interesting for yourself and your friends and family, too. Make running only one aspect of your rich and rewarding life.

**RUN FUNCTIONALLY:** It's really tough to fit everything in and to avoid the feeling that you only have time for work and running. So save time and run to work or run home, or both! Free up some evenings. If you drive to work, park 3 miles away and run the last bit. If you get the bus or train, miss some stops and run the rest. Run to do some shopping, run to the library, run to the post office, or run while your kids bike.

**DENY YOUR BODY RUNNING FOR A FEW DAYS:** To make yourself want to run, stop doing it temporarily. Rest, take a couple of days off, and do something completely different. Miss it; crave it. Deny your body the feelings that come with running. That way, when you come back, you really want to run and are desperate to go.

**RUN AS A TOURIST:** When you travel, open your eyes and really take in the surroundings. Look for things that other tourists won't see, the real

133

life, the heartbeat of the city. Running is the best tourist pass you can have, and you are lucky to have it.

**USE RUNNING TO SOLVE OTHER ISSUES IN YOUR LIFE:** If you're feeling confused, go for a run and really think where that confusion comes from; solve that problem. Run cathartically.

## DEAR KARA

**I've been stressed lately. Work. Kids. Husband time. Me time. I don't have enough time for any of it and I feel like I'm doing everything badly. Do you have any advice?**

It sounds like you have a lot going on and it is impossible to be super at everything in life. Take the time to get out for a run and reflect on all of the things that you are doing right. I'm sure if you think about it, you'll see that you are doing a lot of things right. Focus on those, take deep breaths, and forgive yourself for not being perfect.

**TRY TO BE COMFORTABLE WITH ROTATING PRIORITIES:** Staying in balance doesn't necessarily mean your priorities are and always will be in the same order. By occasionally rotating priorities, you can give your very best to whichever part of your life stands at the top of your list at any one time. And there's no reason that running can't be at the top of that list sometimes, such as when you're approaching a big race for which you have trained for months!

**MAKE DEALS; DO SOME HORSE TRADING:** Maintaining your priorities isn't always easy. Sometimes it takes negotiation, which is fine! For example, occasionally you may need to make deals with your spouse or significant other in order to fulfill your running goals. You might tell your husband: "I'd like to train hard for a marathon this fall, so I'm going to have to put extra time into my running, especially my long runs on Sunday. Can I ask you to take over some of my responsibilities at home? After my marathon, I'll take some of the load off you and give you a break." It's no problem if you talk about it and agree on things up front.

**DON'T WASTE TIME:** As pressed for time as we all are, most of us still manage to waste time each day. Hey, we're human. Don't beat yourself up about it too much. But to have as much time as possible for your priorities each day, it helps to find the waste and trim it. The biggest time waster in my life is the computer. E-mail and the Internet have a way of sucking me in. Yep, I innocently sit down to answer a few messages and catch up on the news of the day, and before I know it an hour has flown by. Sometimes more. At least that's what used to happen before I set a self-imposed limit of 30 minutes of computer time in the morning, and that's it. Between 8 and 8:30 each day, I give myself the freedom to send as many messages and visit as many websites as I want. But when that half hour is up, I shut down the computer and head out to practice. Try it out. Pick a reasonable time limit, choose a time of day that works best, then stick to it.

# DEAR KARA

**I've been crazy busy the last year with my job and my two young children. I'm trying to keep the running going as much as ever, but it's getting tougher, and I resent that I'm being forced to choose between running and my other priorities. What can I do?**

Life is tough and busy. You have children and a job; you are full-time every-thing! I would encourage you to keep up your sanity time. Ask your husband, neighbor, or friend to watch the kids once a week for an hour while you run. If you have to cut back on your runs here and there, that's okay. But you need to take time for you. If you sacrifice your running, you will be resentful. Talk to other people in your life about how you feel. You might find that they can help out so that you can get a run in.

**REMEMBER THAT THERE'S A DIFFERENCE BETWEEN WASTING TIME AND RELAX-ING:** Goodness knows you can always use more of the latter, right? Making time to relax will keep you happier and will also help you perform better during the rest of the day, including on your runs. This might sound crazy, but I schedule my relaxation time just like I do everything else. Between 8 and 10 each evening, Adam and I just sit, watch television, talk, and enjoy each other. It's my favorite part of the day, but no matter how much fun I'm having, when the clock says 10, we go to bed so that we get a good night's sleep and are ready for the next day.

**CREATE A ROUTINE THAT WORKS FOR YOU:** Some people equate routine with boredom or being in a rut, but a routine doesn't have to be that way. Anyone who goes to school or works has to have a routine. The key is to be proactive about it, rather than have it imposed on you. Every day is pretty much the same for me, but I always look forward to almost every part of it, because my routine wasn't forced on me—I chose it! Choose yours, too.

# DEAR KARA

**My husband and I both run, but I'm a lot faster then he is. He says it doesn't bother him, but it would bother me if I were him. What can I do?** Don't obsess over it! You are both runners enjoying the sport. He says it doesn't bother him, so it probably doesn't. He obviously enjoys running for different reasons than being fast. There is nothing wrong with that. Stop worrying about it.

**GIVE OF YOURSELF:** I believe that a truly balanced life includes helping others. To me it's not just a responsibility; it's a personal need that is easy to overlook these days. Helping others feels good and benefits the giver as much as it does the recipient. It's part of the balanced life that enables you to give your best in everything you do, including running.

**PICK WHAT FEELS RIGHT FOR YOU:** Try not to think of helping others as *one more thing* you have to squeeze into an already hectic schedule. There are a million ways to give, so choose one that comes naturally to you and doesn't feel like a burden. My favorite way of helping others is to speak to kids, whether that's student groups, running groups, or clubs. I simply try to share my success in running in hopes of inspiring boys and (especially) girls to aim high in their own lives, whether that's through running or something completely different.

**AVOID REGRET:** If you were taken from Earth tomorrow, would you leave behind any regrets? Hopefully not. But if you know you would, do something about it now. Having regrets is a sure sign that your life is not as balanced as it could be. I always consider the potential for regrets when I make big decisions, such as when I decided to stick with running during the awful and drawn-out period when I was injured so much after college. That's a decision I certainly don't regret!

## DEAR KARA

**Several of my girlfriends take their toddlers for runs in their baby strollers, but I really don't want to do this. They keep asking me about it. I feel like running is my time, not my baby's time. Am I awful for thinking this? I am feeling guilty about it.**

Don't feel guilty about this. While I will occasionally run with my son, 99 percent of the time I won't. Running is something I do for myself; it is my own time. And to run correctly, I need to take my time. I don't want to be rushed or to have to be pushing something or to have to keep checking on someone else. If you enjoy running with your child, then that is wonderful. If you don't, it is perfectly okay. Don't feel guilty about it at all. We all deserve a break from our children!

**PICK ONE NEW THING TO WORK ON EVERY FEW MONTHS:** You can't change everything at once—which doesn't stop some of us from trying. Every three to six months, pick one big thing to focus on and improve. This could be dietary (more soy!), it could be a lifestyle matter (getting consistent sleep), or it could be more directly running related (like adding once-a-week hill running). Your choice.

**HELP SOMEONE ELSE BECOME A RUNNER:** Talk about rewarding—this feels so good. Probably the best way to do this is to (1) give your person a copy of this book and (2) volunteer to run with him or her on the first couple of runs. Take it slow, take it easy, and take plenty of walk breaks.

**LOBBY (DIPLOMATICALLY) FOR BETTER WORKOUT FACILITIES AT WORK:** If you'd prefer to do some of your running during your lunch break (lots of good reasons to do this, by the way) but your workplace doesn't have adequate facilities, mention it to your supervisor or the HR department. Countless companies across the United States are getting with the program and realizing that a fit, healthy employee is a happier, more productive employee. There's all sorts of reliable data that proves this, which you can show the key people at work if need be.

## COACH SALAZAR ON FINDING BALANCE

*There was a time during his elite running days when my coach, Alberto Salazar, was not at all balanced. In fact, by his own admission, he was clearly unbalanced. He was a runner who, if he didn't think 120 miles a week was enough, would do 160. If he didn't think 160 was enough, he'd do 200 (daily average: 28.5 miles). Nothing mattered except to get faster. Known for his laser training focus and take-no-prisoners racing style, Salazar once pushed himself so hard in a race in the heat that he had to be thrown into an ice bath afterward to bring down his soaring body temperature. He survived—after getting last rites.*

*Based on his experiences as Salazar the Runner, Salazar the Coach is in a unique position to talk about the importance of balancing running with all other aspects of your life. It's probably the most important thing he emphasizes to me and the other runners at the Nike Oregon Project. Yes, he has changed a lot. His thoughts:*

**DON'T GIVE RUNNING THE SHORT END OF THE STICK:** First of all, achieving balance is not necessarily doing less running. To be the best runner you can be, you have to do the maximum you can handle. You just need to have other important things in your life as well, such as family, faith, hobbies, and so on.

**BUT KEEP IT IN ITS PLACE:** In fact, those other factors have to be *more* important than running, even for people at Kara's level. As long as you always remember that, even when you're training as hard as you possibly can, you'll be able to maintain balance.

**BE CAREFUL WHAT YOU WISH FOR:** If a runner wants to run with the Nike Oregon Project team and says running is 100 percent the most important thing in the world to her, and really believes that, I can confidently predict that she is going to have short-term success in the sport. She may be incredibly successful, but it won't last long.

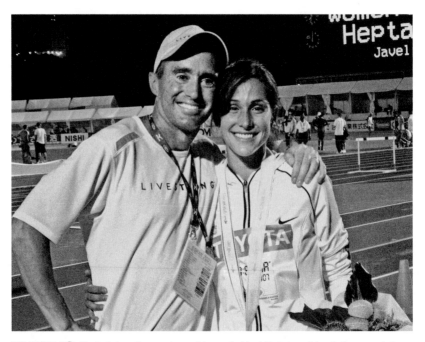

**BALANCING ACT:** Alberto Salazar the runner wasn't known for his ability to keep things in the proper balance. Alberto Salazar the coach makes this a top priority with his runners, including me.

**STAY BALANCED FOR LONG-TERM SUCCESS:** If a runner can stay grounded and surround herself with important things that she cares about, the lows will be less low and the highs will be less high—and I think that's healthy. And chances are, that person is going to have a long and successful career.

## A Day in the Life of . . . Me

If my typical day looks organized, that's because it is. I function best with a regular routine. It may not look fun to you, but it is! I look forward to everything I do each day. Okay, some occasional exceptions, like really tough workouts, but they pass quickly. Here's a normal day for me.

| | |
|---|---|
| 8:00 | Get up and nurse Colt, have coffee and breakfast, go on computer for e-mail, news, etc. |
| 9:25 | Drop Colt off with sitter, head to Nike campus |
| 9:45 | Start warm-up, run, drills, stretching, strides |
| 10:30 | Get spikes on for track session with Coach Alberto |
| 11:30 | Cool down, hurdle drills, stretch |
| 12:30 | Protein shake at gym, then strength train |
| 1:30 | Pick up Colt, head home |
| 2:00 | Eat lunch, catch up on work or read |
| 2:30–3:30 | Get massage |
| 3:45–5:00 | Nap with Colt (yay!) |
| 5:00 | Have a snack, relax, play with Colt |
| 5:30–7:00 | Do second run, plus exercises |
| 7:30 | Make dinner |
| 8:00 | Eat with Adam and Colt |
| 8:45 | Feed Colt and put him down for bed |
| 9:00 | While watching TV with Adam, do stretching routine |
| 10:00 | Start getting ready for bed, read |
| 11:00 | Lights out |

# CHAPTER 6

# FOOD, NUTRITION, AND WEIGHT CONTROL

never thought a thing about my weight all the way through high school and college. I pretty much ate whatever I wanted and never gained weight. Those days ended not long after I graduated from CU. In a few short months I gained 30 pounds and became overweight and unhappy with my body for the first time in my life. This was my first taste of an experience that is all too familiar to a majority of women, including many runners. Fortunately, I found a way to get rid of the extra weight. It did not happen quickly or easily, but it happened. And in the process of shedding all that extra weight, I learned a lot about the weight management techniques that really work and those that do not.

My problems started with another injury. During my junior year at CU, I traveled with my team to Eugene, Oregon, to race. The day after the race, a few of us went for a long run on one of the beautiful wooded trails that have been the regular training grounds for so many great runners from the University of Oregon, from Steve Prefontaine to my current coach, Alberto Salazar. Klutz that I am, I tripped over a root and fell to the ground, my right knee landing smack on the only stone visible on the entire trail.

It hurt like hell. I took a week off. When I resumed running, the knee felt a lot better. Not completely better, though. It became sore at unpredictable times for a while afterward. The problem worsened during my last cross-country season, but fortunately it did not derail my march toward winning the national championship. After that race I skipped the indoor track season once again to heal. But as I ramped up my training in preparation for my final season of collegiate running in the spring, the pain returned, this time worse than ever.

I did my best to push through the problem, but I was really running on one leg. What was meant to be my triumphant final race as a Colorado Buffalo was anything but that—I finished seventh in the NCAA Championships 5,000m, a race I had won the previous year. An MRI performed soon afterward revealed that I had a lingering stress fracture in my kneecap from that darn rock I'd hit the previous year, as well as severe chondromalacia in the same knee. Chondromalacia is basically chewed-up cartilage—a condition that afflicts the knees of many runners (or that many runners inflict on their knees!). I was also diagnosed with tendinitis in the patellar tendon of that knee. A real triple whammy. My orthopedist recommended surgery to file down my fissured knee cartilage—a serious procedure that would take me out for the whole summer. Having just signed a professional contract with Nike, I was eager to get started on my career, so I decided to pass on the operation and instead rest for a few weeks to see if that fixed the problem.

Every few days I would test the knee with some slow strides in hopes of feeling a little less soreness, and each time I was disappointed. August came around and still I could neither run nor seriously cross-train. I went in for another MRI. It confirmed what I already knew: the damage remained. So we scheduled surgery for October, after Adam and I got back from a trip to Fiji.

That's right: our honeymoon! Adam and I had planned a wedding

143

on September 16 in Lyons, Colorado. In the weeks leading up to the big event, I found myself in the position of many brides-to-be: needing to lose weight to fit into my wedding dress and look presentable on the most important day of my life. Many weeks of inactivity had caused extra pounds to accumulate on my body for the first time ever. Since I was already doomed to go under the knife, I went ahead and ran and cross-trained like crazy, toughing out the pain to get back down to my normal dress size.

The flight home from Fiji brought me to a bad new reality. When the surgeon opened up my knee, he discovered that chondromalacia was the least of my problems. A section of my patellar tendon had literally died because of chronic inflammation of the tissue. He had to remove all of the dead tissue, leaving only three-quarters of the tendon behind. My rehabilitation from this unexpectedly invasive procedure would take much longer than expected. For a while I would be almost completely unable to do any form of exercise.

And then I went home. The distractions of travel (I had spent much of the summer following Adam around Europe from track meet to track meet) and the wedding were behind us. Adam and I began our life together as husband-and-wife professional runners, but I couldn't run or do much of anything else. Unable to train and without school to entertain me, I fell into a bottomless pit of boredom. Each day stretched endlessly before me with almost nothing to fill it. When Adam rolled out of bed in the morning to get ready for his first run, I tried my best to fall back asleep and stay asleep as long as possible. On a good day I was still in bed when Adam came back at eleven. On most days he found me sitting in front of the television, watching soap operas without interest, eating entire bowls of cashews and candy corn. That's right: cashews and candy corn.

I felt robbed of any purpose or usefulness. This period of involuntarily inactivity had taken me completely off guard and I had no Plan B. I had envisioned my life as a professional runner being filled with training, travel, racing, and time with Adam. Now I had only Adam, and he still had his training and racing. I had nothing. A dark cloud settled over my head and stayed there.

In a word, I became depressed, and as it does for a lot of women, depression made me eat. It became a vicious circle: depression led to overeating, which made me even more depressed, which in turn made me eat even more. I would wolf down an entire box of sugary cereal in front of the television in the middle of the morning, and then I would feel guilty about it and think: What am I doing? I can't even work this off! Then I would think: Well, I'm already too far gone, so I might as well keep eating. And then I would eat some more. It was completely self-defeating.

I got some relief in February, four months after the surgery, when my doctor gave me permission to start doing nonimpact exercise. Adam and I had an elliptical trainer at home and I went at it like an addict, working out for an hour in the morning and another hour in the afternoon in a desperate effort to get my body back. I went at it so aggressively that I fractured my right femur on that stupid machine. Only one person in the history of the world has ever fractured a femur on an elliptical trainer, and that person is me.

After looking at the X-ray, my baffled doctor told me that I was now forbidden to do any form of exercise involving my legs for another six weeks. "If you're not careful, I'll have to put a rod in your leg and your running career will be over," he said sternly.

As you might imagine, I quickly regained the little weight I had lost and added a whole lot more.

To this day I remain an emotional eater. When I am under a lot of stress, I crave sweets and starches and lots of them. It drives me crazy that I am such a puppet to my emotions. Breaking the strings completely is impossible. I am who I am. But I have found that simply recognizing my emotional eating saves me from the worst excesses during stressful and unhappy times. I will catch myself heading out the door to drive down to the bakery for some brownies and say, "Hold on, Kara: *Why* do you want those brownies?" If it's because of an emotional trigger, I am sometimes—not always, but sometimes—able to turn around and find some other outlet, like calling a friend or cooking something healthy.

This is a big change from that postsurgery period when I said yes to every temptation. Six months after my wedding day, I weighed 30 pounds more than when Adam had promised to stick with me for better or worse. I felt bad about letting myself go so quickly. For his own sake, Adam could not have been happy about the transformation my body had undergone, but he knew that getting on a female runner's case about her weight was like dancing in a minefield. At the same time, he also knew that I needed help. So he stayed quiet most of the time, but every once in a while he would gently say something like, "Honey, maybe you should take it a little easy on the candy corn for a while." He's so adorable!

I became ashamed of how I looked—so ashamed that I left home as seldom as possible. But sometimes I had no choice but to venture into public. Even though I was injured, Nike asked me to make an appearance at the 2001 Foot Locker Cross Country Championship. I felt terribly uncomfortable the whole time I was there, because everyone around me looked really fit and I was overweight and couldn't hide it. My brother-in-law was competing in the race that year and noticed my weight gain. He later told me that when he first saw me there he wondered, Who's the shot putter? before recognizing me.

Nobody actually said anything to me about my appearance, but their bodies said enough. They looked lean, healthy, and fast. I did not. At the grocery store or the mall, I could fit in and feel less self-conscious, but around other runners I stood out and was hyperaware of my soft appearance. I look sad in the photographs taken during that time. My eyes seemed to say: I know I have an issue right now and I don't know what to do about it!

Again, my weight was only a symptom of the real problem, which was depression compounded by boredom. Fittingly, I started on the road toward correcting my weight problem by addressing the depression and boredom. The thing that spurred me into action was the guilt I felt about being such dead weight in my marriage. Adam did everything for both of us, including all the cooking. I decided that I needed to take some of the burden off his shoulders, and learning how to cook seemed like a sensible way to do that.

I went to the bookstore and bought a Betty Crocker cookbook. It was very basic because basic was all I could handle. I mastered that and then bought a book of stir-fry recipes, and then a book on vegetables.

My new infatuation with the kitchen was more about the preparation of the food and making something that tasted good than it was about better nutrition and losing weight. I learned to appreciate the process, from shopping for quality ingredients to choosing a recipe to try to making it all come together in the kitchen to enjoying it (or not!) with Adam. In fact, it was about filling time as much as anything else. The more time it took, the better. I liked recipes that took an hour to make. I liked recipes that took three hours even more.

Not everything came out well. Some dishes came out tasting terrible; others came out flavorless. I made fajitas that tasted like sugar. I spent hours making an Italian chicken dish that was like sawdust on the tongue. Adam had little choice but to eat everything and he never complained. No matter what I made or how it turned out, he said the same thing: "It's really good!" I had to study his eyes and the shape of his mouth to discern which meals he truly enjoyed and which he forced down for the sake of encouraging me.

I stayed encouraged. If a recipe came out badly I crossed it off the list and moved on. I was enjoying the process and my skills were improving day by day, so I ploughed ahead. The wholesomeness of the things I made was at first a side benefit that I came to appreciate more and more as time passed. Before my cooking made any difference in my weight, it washed away the guilt that eating badly caused me. Instead of eating an entire box of cereal by myself and then wishing I hadn't, I would share with Adam a hot, tasty meal made with fresh ingredients. I felt good about it.

148

The decision to learn how to cook is one of the better decisions I have made. It transformed my relationship to food. Before I learned how to cook, food controlled me. I just ate whatever was easy and tasted good. Learning to cook put me in control of the food I ate. It made me think about the quality of the ingredients I bought, the nutritional balance of the meals I prepared, and even the portion sizes I served myself. Eating became more about savoring flavors and appreciating my handiwork and less about filling my stomach.

I don't think it's merely coincidental that the decline in home cooking paralleled the rise in overweight and obesity in our society. People tend to eat healthier and eat less when they cook for themselves. A lot of women and men resist cooking today because they were never taught how to do it, so the kitchen intimidates them, and they've convinced themselves that they don't have time to cook. It takes a little courage and resolve to push through these barriers and get started, but if you do, I think you will soon find yourself wondering what the big deal was and why you waited so long, which is precisely what happened to me. You can make a tasty, healthy dinner at home in less than thirty minutes, or about as long as it takes to run out and grab takeout and not much longer than it takes to heat up something boxed or canned.

Around this time, I started working with sports nutritionist Dan Bernadot, which helped me a lot. (You will get some of his wisdom in the advice section of this chapter.) It was actually one of the best things I've ever done for my health and wellness. Any woman who is struggling to manage her weight would be well advised to do the same. Most of us behave as our own worst enemies when we're trying to lose weight. We make the same common mistakes such as trying to starve our way thinner, which only sabotages our efforts by slowing our metabolism. We get stuck in patterns of emotional eating that we can't get out of. And we are held back by our own ignorance about nutrition.

A good nutritionist can help you with all of these things. Properly educated about nutrition and weight management, your nutritionist can pass that education along to you—not only telling you what to do and what not to do, but equipping you with tools and information that enable you to nourish yourself correctly long after you've stopped working with him or her. Also, like a running coach, a nutritionist offers an objective external perspective that can help you keep your emotions from derailing your weight-management efforts.

Hiring a nutritionist is not as expensive as you might think. Most work for reasonable hourly rates and offer affordable package deals for certain types of services. As in any service profession, some nutritionists are better than others. Anyone can call himself a nutritionist without any formal training or certification, so seek out those who have the better credentials, such as registered dietitians. If you are a competitive runner, I suggest you work with a certified sports nutritionist. General nutritionists aren't always well trained in the needs of serious athletes.

In the end, learning to cook and learning about nutrition from Dan got me going in the right direction with my eating and my weight, but it was my return to regular training—including strength training—that brought me all the way back. Regular exercise is just so important for weight control. To this day, my weight will occasionally fluctuate. This scares me a little, but only a little. I know that a certain amount of weight fluctuation over the course of the year is normal and unavoidable for any serious runner. And having learned all I did through my first battle with being overweight, I know that I have the power to always remain the master of my body.

I'm sure the following advice will help you stay on track with your nutrition and weight-control goals.

FOOD, NUTRITION, AND WEIGHT CONTROL

# CAN'T-FAIL TIPS AND PLANS TO HELP YOU EAT RIGHT, CONTROL YOUR WEIGHT, AND STAY ENERGIZED ON EVERY RUN

Many American women have an adversarial relationship with food. Among women runners, it's more like war.

Many women runners think that if they could just lose a little more weight, they'd be faster. Sure, this is true sometimes, if they're carrying a lot of extra pounds. But too many women don't know when to switch that thinking off. They don't recognize when this thought process becomes counterproductive and even dangerous.

Making this worse, this "if I could just lose weight, I'd be fine" thinking often morphs into a "food is bad" mentality. And for runners especially, food is not bad. Food is good. Food is absolutely essential for providing the energy you need to run and do everything else you do each day.

My own relationship with food has been a bit rocky in the past—I don't deny that. But I've learned a lot about myself, and about food and nutrition as well, and I think I'm in a really good place now. I'm excited about all the great advice in this chapter. It comes from some of the country's leading sports nutritionists and weight-control experts.

**BE OKAY WITH HEALTHY FATS:** Healthy fats—namely the unsaturated fats in plant foods—are as important to me as carbohydrates and protein. Many runners believe that all fat is bad, but I learned long ago that fat is a critical part of a healthy diet. It must be the right fat (and not too much of it). I'm talking about such sources as olive oil and avocados, not steak gristle!

**TRY TO MAKE YOUR MEALS WELL ROUNDED:** I don't worry too much about getting percentages of this or that type of macronutrient (carbohydrates, fat, and protein). I just try to combine foods that are good sources of each. I have found that including all three macronutrients in each meal keeps my appetite under control and keeps my energy level steady throughout the day.

**EAT BREAKFAST EVERY DAY:** You've probably heard this healthy eating and weight-control tip before, and it's a great one. It's good to do this so that you don't start your day hungry—only to spend the rest of the day catching up by eating whatever comes in front of your face. As soon as I wake up, I make myself breakfast and sit down in front of the computer to eat (not optimal, I know, but better than eating on the go). For me it's usually oatmeal or—ready for this?—whole wheat toast with cheese spread. I also include a piece of fruit and usually almonds (read: healthy fat), along with coffee. Worldwide eating

## DEAR KARA

**Are there any vitamins or supplements I should take as a woman runner? Do you take any?**
As a women runner I think it is a good idea to take extra calcium and extra iron. This will help prevent any stress fractures or anemia. Along with a good multivitamin, this should cover your bases.

surveys have shown that people who eat breakfast maintain healthier body weights compared to those who skip breakfast.

**BE MINDFUL ABOUT IRON:** As a woman runner, you are more prone to low iron than male runners. If your workouts and/or races suddenly drop off a cliff in terms of performance, that's a clear sign that you may need a simple blood test for iron. Women sometimes don't get enough iron in their diets (shying away from red meat is a frequent cause), and they lose iron due to their monthly cycle.

## DEAR KARA

**I thought running was going to help me lose weight, but so far it hasn't. I've been running 15 miles a week for about four months. Do I have to run more? Eat less? Both?**

This is tricky. It could be a combination of both. Fifteen miles a week might not be quite as challenging as it was for your body at first. You might need to keep bumping it up. You also might need to eat less. Even with running, if you aren't burning more calories than you are putting in, you won't lose weight. Try not to obsess about the scale. How do you feel? Do your clothes fit better? Sometimes you don't lose weight because you are gaining muscle, which weighs more than fat. When this happens, you might not see the scale move, but your clothes will fit better.

**"GRAZE" WITH SMALLER MEALS:** Large meals may contain the carbohydrate and protein you need to satisfy your muscular and fuel needs, but because of all the calories you're taking in at the same time, these meals tend to be fat producing. So that large, high-carbohydrate pasta meal before the race that you thought was giving your muscles a glycogen advantage may actually be a high-fat meal in disguise. Eating the

153

same amount in smaller meals more frequently is a much more effective strategy.

**GET USED TO SNACKING:** Eating a small snack between meals that provides 150 to 250 calories will help you sustain blood sugar, keep your central nervous system working well, and help you avoid breaking down muscle to supply the needed fuel for the brain. Never go longer than three hours without something to eat.

**TAKE IN CALORIES SOON AFTER RUNNING FOR OPTIMAL RECOVERY:** Plan to consume 400 to 500 calories immediately after training if possible, and another 400 to 500 calories about one to two hours after that. The reason? Glycogen synthetase, the enzyme that captures glucose to store it as glycogen, is at its peak immediately after training.

**GET TIMELY WITH YOUR EATING AND EXERCISE:** Having to constantly ratchet down your food intake to keep from gaining weight is a sign that energy intake and energy requirement are not well matched. Make a simple graph that estimates the times of day you are expending the most and least energy. On the same graph, plot out when you are consuming the most and least energy. The peaks in energy intake should closely match the peaks in energy expenditure, *but* they should be about two to three hours earlier. Alternatively, you can go to NutriTiming.com to do this scientifically.

**TRY NOT TO WRITE OFF ENTIRE FOOD CATEGORIES:** Women runners can be prone to avoiding whole categories of foods by labeling them good, bad, or fattening. Some runners, for instance, give carbohydrates the label of fattening, even though this is far and away the most important macronutrient for you and your running. Unfortunately, this habit almost guarantees malnutrition and poor athletic performance. All foods can be fattening if you consume too much of them at one time. By spreading out your food intake and consuming smaller meals, you'll avoid the hormonal and endocrine shifts that encourage muscle loss and fat gain.

**BEWARE OF HIGH PROTEIN:** Stress fractures can actually be a signal that your protein intake is too high, as excess protein increases calcium loss in the urine. Generally speaking, if you get a stress fracture, that's a good time to seriously evaluate if your training regimen and nutrition plan are appropriately matched.

**SUPPLEMENT YOUR EATING WHEN NEEDED:** For various reasons, you may not be getting certain nutrients you need just from the foods you eat. Supplementation may be necessary. Here are three important supplements:

- **Calcium:** Seven out of ten women do not get enough calcium through their diet alone. Younger women need 1,000 mg of calcium per day; postmenopausal women need 1,500 mg. Either try for three to four servings per day of milk or calcium-fortified beverages, or take a calcium supplement to keep your bones strong. Remember, chocolate milk is a great recovery food after your long runs! If you can't get enough calcium in your diet, you may need to take a supplement.
- **Vitamin D:** Along with calcium, you need vitamin D for strong bones and for good health. The body actually needs vitamin D to absorb calcium. Most experts are now recommending 1,000 IU per day. Vitamin D is found naturally in few foods, such as salmon, and is added to fortified milk and diary products. As with calcium, you may need to take a supplement if you don't get enough in your diet.
- **Fish oil:** Omega-3 fatty acids are important for helping you recover from your runs, and they're vital for heart and brain health. If you don't eat 6 ounces of fatty fish per week, you need to supplement with 600 to 1,000 mg per day.

**EAT PLENTY DURING YOUR TRAINING BUILDUP FOR A RACE:** During these times, your food intake must support your increased nutritional needs for muscle repair and recovery, and endurance expansion. This is not the

## ON THE CONTRARY

I know some runners worry a lot about carbo-loading, but I've found that if I've been eating a balanced diet, there is no need to gorge myself with huge portions of pasta the days leading up to a race. In fact, the shorter the race, the more I worry about getting some good protein in the night before.

A lot of people worry about not eating dessert or drinking alcohol the night before a race. I don't. If I feel like a glass of wine or a cookie, I have it. It won't hurt my performance.

time to restrict food with the hope of losing body fat, as you'll increase your risk of illness and injury. Your best strategy is to eat enough food to increase your energy, raise your training, build muscle, and then you can burn fat during the race. Eat simple, wholesome foods as often as possible, such as fresh and dried fruit, nuts, organic mozzarella cheese sticks, yogurt, soy chips, turkey or tuna jerky, hard-boiled eggs, cut-up vegetables, edamame, peanut butter and jelly (perhaps with apple butter instead of jelly) on sprouted wheat bread, even a turkey sandwich. While protein energy bars are not my favorite choice, they are convenient. Look for brands that offer at least 10 grams of protein, real fruit and nuts, and no fractionated oils.

**FUEL YOUR MUSCLES AND FEED YOUR BRAIN:** Combine protein and carbohydrates at each meal and snack, and you will raise your muscle fuel and your mood at the same time. The good-mood combo of protein plus carbohydrates raises serotonin levels in the brain and enhances muscle refueling, recovery, and growth. Milk is an ideal feel-great food, combining quickly digested whey protein with lactose, a natural carbohydrate. Also helpful to serotonin production and physical activity is the vitamin D you get in fortified milk.

**PUT YOUR CARBOHYDRATES TO WORK FOR YOU:** Just because you burn a lot of calories during running doesn't mean that it's time to load up on sugar. Rather:

- Eat whole foods that are rich in carbohydrates for every meal, including whole fruits and vegetables, and whole grains and beans.
- Choose carbohydrate-rich beverages that are low in added sugars and high in nutrient value, such as nonfat or low-fat milk, 100% fruit and vegetable juice, and other beverages with no or very low amounts of added sugar.

**EAT AN EGG YOLK A DAY:** Choline, the B vitamin found in large amounts in egg yolks, is half of the neurotransmitter compound called acetyl-

157

# Get Plenty of Anti-Inflammatory Foods

One of the side effects of being a runner is inflammation inside your body. Certain foods can help you lower inflammation, whereas others can actually exacerbate it. Get plenty of anti-inflammatory foods, and minimize your intake of pro-inflammatory foods.

| Anti-inflammatory Foods | Pro-inflammatory Foods |
|---|---|
| Apples | Safflower oil |
| Citrus fruits and juices | Corn oil |
| Fatty fish | Sesame oil |
| Ginger | Margarine |
| Green beans | Partially hydrogenated oils |
| Kale | Shortening |
| Nuts | Sugars and refined starches in high |
| Olives | amounts |
| Olive oil (extra-virgin) | |
| Onions | |
| Pineapples | |
| Pomegranates | |
| Prunes | |
| Turmeric | |
| Vegetable oils | |
| Wheat germ | |

choline. The most abundant neurotransmitter in the body, acetylcholine is responsible for every thought and every movement that you have. Phosphatidylcholine and phosphatidylserine, which are also found in egg yolks, create the channels in brain cell membrane to allow nutrients to pass into the cell and toxins to pass out. Yet on average, Americans only get about a third of their daily need for choline. Why? Because medical authorities mistakenly associated eating eggs with elevated blood cholesterol decades ago. Several studies have now shown that an egg yolk a day does not raise cholesterol levels in healthy individuals. So try this: Hard boil seven eggs at the beginning of the week and refrigerate them for an easy and tasty egg for breakfast or a snack each day. You will feel the difference.

## DEAR KARA

**Do you have a favorite "girl food" that you depend on?**
I do like the lighter-calorie sport drinks that are geared more toward women. I like to take a sport drink during and after exercise, but I don't want to chug down 200 to 400 calories in doing so. The lighter half-calorie versions are great. You get the same benefit but without the extra calories.

**TRY CAFFEINE BEFORE A RUN TO MAKE IT EASIER:** That's right—put caffeine to work for you by consuming it before exercise, as it can lower your perception of how hard you're working. Therefore, you'll be able to train harder for a longer period before you notice that you're working so hard. To achieve this effect, you need about 1.3 mg per pound of body weight. So if you weigh 140 pounds, you need about 182 mg of caffeine to get a performance-enhancing benefit. An average 8-ounce cup of brewed coffee contains 80–100 mg of caffeine, and 8 ounces of black tea contains around 50 mg.

**GET ENOUGH HIGH-PERFORMANCE FATS!** There's no reason to be fat phobic. Sixty percent of the mass of your brain is fat. No surprise then that diets that include less than 25 percent of calories from fat can lower coping skills and increase feelings of anxiety and frustration. Choose high-performance fats from fish, extra-virgin olive oil, olives, nuts, avocados, nut butters, and canola and grapeseed oils. Try to include

159

them at all meals and snacks, except in the hours before you run, when they can slow digestion.

**DRINK YOUR RECOVERY SHAKE BEFORE YOU DO ANYTHING ELSE:** If you change only one thing in your diet as a runner, drink a recovery shake right after each run, *then* shower and get dressed. It will make a noticeable difference in how you feel for the rest of the day, how well you recover, and how hard you train on successive days. The key is combining protein (whey protein is ideal) with carbohydrate within 15 to 30 minutes after you finish your run. If you can't have a shake or smoothie, go for chocolate milk. Then follow that with a meal within two hours to keep the muscle-recovery fires burning.

**STAY WELL HYDRATED ALL DAY:** Nothing will deplete your physical and mental performance faster than dehydration. Along with all the other fluids you take in throughout the day (milk, 100% fruit juice, coffee, tea, etc.), drink at least 40 to 48 ounces of water. Research shows that people who drink at least this amount of water each day, versus those who drink 16 ounces or less, have a significantly lower risk of cancers of the urinary tract, colon, and possibly breast, along with a lower risk of heart attack, stroke, and mitral valve prolapse. Be in the habit of drinking 16 ounces of fluid before exercise, and 4 to 8 ounces of fluid every 15 to 20 minutes during exercise. After exercise, replace each pound you lose by sweating with 20 to 24 ounces of fluid.

**ALLOW AT LEAST TWO HOURS TO DIGEST YOUR MEAL BEFORE A RUN OR RACE:** Your muscles require more blood during running than they do at rest, so your stomach may not get the normal blood flow needed for digestion. The food in your stomach will stay there longer, causing discomfort or even cramping.

**BE CAREFUL ABOUT SUGARY FOODS:** Before a run or race, it's important to limit foods such as soft drinks, jelly beans, maple syrup, and sugary ce-

## DEAR KARA

I sometimes see overweight, sedentary women and almost get angry with them for it. I mean, how can they get like that?! I can't help feeling this way. Any thoughts?

Not everyone has an incredible athletic work ethic. You never know what someone has been through. Maybe you are seeing someone who gained weight while pregnant, had difficulty losing the weight, and is now embarrassed to get out and exercise. Don't judge anybody. Be a positive example. Don't ever discourage someone from trying to better their life and health.

real. Most runners will be fine with these foods, but occasionally they cause symptoms of rebound hypoglycemia such as light-headedness and fatigue.

**DON'T USE ALCOHOL TO CARBO-LOAD (IT DOESN'T WORK):** Alcohol is not a good source of carbohydrates. A standard 12-ounce bottle of beer contains only 14 grams (or 56 calories) of carbohydrates, whereas a 12-ounce can of soda provides 40 grams (160 calories). Therefore, a beer the night before a race or long run is fine, but combine it with a thick-crust pizza or other carbohydrate-rich foods.

**GO WITH NATURAL CARBOHYDRATES TO GAIN ENERGY *AND* NUTRIENTS:** All sources of carbohydrates are not created equal, though most have a similar ability to fuel your muscles. Here's the lowdown:

- Soft drinks provide energizing carbohydrates for the muscles but no vitamins or minerals.
- Sport drinks provide energizing carbohydrates for the muscles but no vitamins or minerals, unless the drink is fortified.

# Your Perfect Day of Eating

Here is a 2,200-calorie, highly nutritious, energy-boosting daylong menu for women runners. To customize the calorie intake level for you, see the substitution ideas at the end of the menu.

This menu's macronutrient breakdown is 55% carbohydrates, 25% protein, and 20% fat, which is optimal for runners. The rationale? Carbohydrates are your muscles' primary fuel source during running. They are also rate-limited nutrients, meaning you can only store approximately 1,800 calories of carbohydrates in the form of muscle glycogen. A high-carbohydrate diet can actually increase that glycogen storage capability, boost energy levels, and improve your running perfomance.

### Breakfast

Kashi Go Lean Crunch with skim milk
*Why:* 1 serving contains 8 grams of protein, 10 grams of fiber.

Kefir, 1 cup
*Why:* This is a probiotic-rich liquid yogurt, and has been shown to improve immune function, which can be compromised in distance runners.

Dried cranberries or cherries, ¼ cup
*Why:* Excellent source of vitamin C and other antioxidants. Runners are prone to upper respiratory tract infections more than other athletes; food sources of vitamin C can be protective.

### Midmorning Snack

Low-fat Greek yogurt, 1 cup
*Why:* This is a higher-protein yogurt—10 to 16 grams of protein per cup versus 5 to 6 grams in most types. Women are prone to not getting enough protein due to greater incidence of vegetarianism.

Soya granules mixed into the yogurt, ⅛ cup serving

*Why:* 11 grams of soy protein and 50 calories. Excellent source of vegetarian protein.

### Lunch

Sandwich of whole wheat bread, 2 slices; or 1 whole wheat wrap

Grilled chicken, turkey, or fish, 3 ounces

Whole-grain mustard and/or reduced-fat salad dressing

Lettuce, tomato, cucumber, sprouts

*Why:* Full of fiber, vitamins C and A, and lycopene. Stuffing sandwiches with vegetables bulks up the entree without bulking up the calories, which appeals to calorie-counting women runners.

Purple seedless grapes, 1 cup

*Why:* High in vitamin C and a cardio-protective antioxidant called resveritrol.

Vegetable soup

*Why:* Broth-based soup is a nutritious, low-calorie food that adds a lot of fiber and vitamins C and A to your diet.

Iced unsweetened green tea

*Why:* Good source of epigallocatechin gallate (EGCG), an antioxidant with antiviral activity, good for boosting immune function.

### Afternoon Snack

Mix of raw vegetables (radishes, carrots, celery, pepper strips)

Hummus, ½ cup

*Why:* You get 6 grams of plant protein, fiber, and vitamin E, a potent cell-protecting antioxidant.

163

## Dinner

Grilled chicken or fish, 4 ounces

Mango salsa, ½ cup
*Why:* Mango is rich in vitamin C.

Steamed broccoli, 1½ cups
*Why:* Contains diindolylmethane, a potent anticancer chemical.

1 medium sweet potato with brown sugar or maple syrup, 2 tablespoons
*Why:* Sweet potatoes are high in beta-carotene, vitamin C, and fiber. Beta-carotene and vitamin C protect cell membranes.

Skim milk, 1 cup
*Why:* 8 grams of high-quality absorbable protein, 300 milligrams of calcium, and a good source of vitamin D.

## Postdinner Snack

Skinny Cow ice cream sandwich

## To Add Extra Calories

*Midmorning snack:* Instead of low-fat Greek yogurt, use full-fat yogurt and mix in ¼ cup of dried blueberries.
*Afternoon snack:* Add 1 cup trail mix (a mixture of almonds, peanuts, walnuts, pecans, dried fruit).
*Breakfast and lunch:* Use 2% milk instead of skim.

## To Reduce Calories

*Midmorning snack:* Skip the soya granules.
*Afternoon snack:* Skip the hummus.

- Fruits, vegetables, and grains provide energizing carbohydrates for the muscles, along with vitamins, minerals, fiber, and phytochemicals—all of which your body needs to function at its best.

**STAY BLAND THE DAY BEFORE YOUR RACE:** Keep away from spicy food the day before and morning of your race. They, along with your nervous stomach, can bring on gastric upset. It's smart to avoid them even if you've tried the foods before.

**HYDRATE APPROPRIATELY DURING YOUR RACE:** If your race distance is a 10K or shorter, you probably don't need to hydrate with sport drinks before or during the race. The carbohydrates in sport drinks aid energy needs in long runs and races. The electrolytes supply minerals lost when you sweat for an extended period. Shorter races don't require extra carbohydrates or electrolytes. Just drink and eat after the race.

**TRY THESE DURING YOUR RACE:** Sport gels, sport blocks, and sport beans are relatively new but effective products for runners in longer races, and some of them even taste good. Just be sure to experiment with them before race day.

## Weight Control

**LIFT TO STAY LEAN:** I'm not sure why it works so well for me, but strength training has an amazing power to lean me out. They say muscle burns more calories than fat and maybe that's the key. Strength training also improves my tone, which makes me *look* leaner, even if I may not actually *be* leaner.

165

**AIM TO TRAIN, NOT TO BURN FAT:** Burning fat gets seriously overhyped in women's health and fitness magazines, and people can get pretty obsessed with it. To me, it's the wrong motivation. I actually don't run

# Your Can't-Fail Prerace Eating Plan

The key to prerace eating is going with low-fiber, carbohydrate-rich food. The carbohydrates optimize your ability to make and store the key muscle fuel, glycogen. Prerace eating begins the day *before* the race.

## The Day Before

**Breakfast** (includes 55% carbohydrates, 25% protein, 20% fat)

Special K cereal, 1½ cups

Skim milk, 1 cup or Greek yogurt, 1 cup

Peach or berries, 1 cup

Orange juice, 1 cup

Banana bread, 1 slice, with peanut butter

**Lunch** (includes 55% carbohydrates, 25% protein, 20% fat)

Medium-sized grilled chicken and mozzarella cheese wrap with lettuce and tomato

Low-fat salad dressing on the wrap, 1 tablespoon

Progresso Hearty Tomato soup, ½ can (9.5 ounces)

Skim milk, 1 cup

**Afternoon Snack**

Golden Delicious apple with 3 tablespoons almond butter

**Dinner** (includes 60% carbohydrates, 20% protein, 20% fat)

Grilled salmon, 4 ounces

White rice, 2 cups (more if your race is a half marathon or marathon)

Steamed broccoli, 1 cup (more if you desire)

Salad containing lettuce or spinach, tomatoes, carrots, mushrooms, and red cabbage

KARA GOUCHER'S RUNNING FOR WOMEN

Low-fat dressing, 3 tablespoons

Dinner roll with 1 teaspoon butter or olive oil

### Optional Late-Night Snack

Pure carbohydrates! Good choices: cheese and crackers or pretzels and
hummus.

*Note:* There's no need to eat if you're not hungry. Your goal is to go to bed having
eaten a high-carbohydrate dinner. If you have a half marathon or marathon, you
deserve a higher-calorie meal but may prefer to have a snack in the evening rather
than eat a large dinner.

## Race Day

Depending on the time of the race, the following rules apply:

- **3 hours before running:** You can eat a real meal that includes a bowl of low-fiber cereal and skim milk or yogurt, *or* a turkey sandwich on white bread or honey wheat bread, 8 ounces of juice or your favorite sport drink, and a banana. At this point, you have time to digest, absorb, and metabolize the food.
- **As you get closer to race time:** Switch to carbohydrate-only snacks. Go for smaller amounts of food that are fiber-free and easy to digest. Never experiment with a new food on race day.
- **Each hour leading up to the race:** Drink 16 ounces of fluid. If the race is short, water is all you need. Otherwise, a sport drink is best.
- **An hour before the race:** Eat four to six animal crackers or two graham crackers for additional carbohydrates.
- **15 to 30 minutes before race time:** Have a packet of your favorite sport gel or good old honey (about ½ oz.) for a last-minute energy boost of pure carbohydrates, which is rapidly absorbed for energy.

or do any other kind of training specifically to burn fat. Everything I do along those lines is to improve my performance. If fat-burning happens at the same time—and I'm sure it does—that's just fine with me. I just don't think fat-burning is a very realistic or motivating goal over the long term, but trying to be the best runner you can be certainly is.

**REMEMBER THAT WEIGHT LOSS WON'T HAPPEN AUTOMATICALLY:** A lot of men and women start running because they think it will help them lose weight. And, in fact, it is one of the best weight-loss weapons around. But as with everything else in your weight-loss arsenal, running can't do it all by itself. You need to control other things at the same time— namely food intake. If you're not creating a regular calorie deficit— that is, expending more calories than you take in—all the running in the world won't bring you weight loss.

**FOCUS ON EATING QUALITY FOODS, NOT ON *DIETING*:** This is an important point, which is to focus on all the great foods you can eat and how much fuel your body needs as a runner. If you're always focusing on restriction—on foods you're not allowed to eat—your weight-control plan is going to fail.

**ENJOY WHOLE GRAINS, FRUIT, AND/OR VEGETABLES WITH EVERY MEAL:** They're loaded with disease-fighting and health-enhancing vitamins, minerals, phytochemicals, and antioxidants. And here's something else. When you start eating, get in the habit of starting with these foods first. Why? The water and fiber in them will fill you up, so you'll naturally end up eating less of the other things on offer, some of which may be higher in sugar, calories, and fat.

**LIMIT REFINED FOODS SUCH AS WHITE BAGELS AND SUGARS:** These foods tend to be low in fiber, so they don't fill you up. Also, they tend to

# Great Weight-Loss Tips from the World's Best Losers

An ongoing study called the National Weight Control Registry (NWCR) is currently tracking more than five thousand women and men who have lost 30 pounds or more and have kept the weight off for at least a year. (Individual weight losses range from 30 to 300 pounds.) These people know how to control their weight.

"By changing my self-talk, I went from thinking that reading in bed was an aerobic activity to running half marathons," says NWCR member Sandra Wright, who lost 100 pounds and has kept it off for five years. "I'm now an active, healthy, energetic woman who loves to exercise," she says. The keys to her success: learning portion control, keeping food records, and getting regular exercise.

## Facts About NWCR Members

- Eighty percent of people in the registry are women; 20 percent are men.
- Members have lost an average of 66 pounds and kept it off for five and a half years.
- Some lost the weight slowly; others did so gradually in as many as fourteen years.

## How did they lose the weight initially?

- Forty-five percent lost the weight on their own; 55 percent did so with help from a program.
- Ninety-four percent increased their physical activity (walking is the most popular form of exercise).
- Ninety-eight percent modified their food intake in some way.

## How do they keep the weight off?

- Most do high levels of activity. Ninety percent say they average 1 hour of exercise daily.
- Most maintain a low-calorie, low-fat eating plan.
- Seventy-eight percent eat breakfast every day.
- Seventy-five percent weigh themselves at least once a week.
- Sixty-two percent watch less than 10 hours of television a week.

jack your blood sugar up and down in no time, and when it goes down, it crashes. At which point you feel hungrier than you did before you ate, and meanwhile you didn't get that many other nutrients either. A lot of the low-carb diets that are still around are all about this idea of getting refined carbohydrates and sugars out of your diet, which is why they occasionally work.

**KEEP TRACK OF YOUR FOOD INTAKE USING A JOURNAL WHEN YOU MAKE HEALTHY CHANGES TO YOUR EATING PLAN:** Try to do this for at least three weeks, which is how long it normally takes to establish new habits. If it's effective and not too much of a pain, keep doing it for as long as you wish. There are lots of downloadable programs that allow you to track your food intake, but a paper journal is probably still the easiest method.

**WEIGH YOURSELF WEEKLY TO HELP TRACK YOUR WEIGHT-CONTROL PROGRESS:** Some women have success weighing themselves more frequently— sometimes every day—but you don't want to become obsessed with it. Once a week is probably best. And yes, weighing yourself does work. It's one of the key weight-control methods used by women in the on-going National Weight Control Registry. Each participant in the registry has maintained at least a 30-pound weight loss for a year or more.

**EXERCISE PORTION CONTROL:** Often, when women meet with a nutrition counselor and are shown the list of foods they can eat each day, they are pleasantly relieved. However, the catch often comes when they learn about portion sizes. It's important to learn portion sizes so that you'll have an immediate sense of how much you're eating. For example, a cup is roughly the size of a baseball. A half cup is the size of a computer mouse. A serving of meat is the size of a deck of cards. And, not to give you the shakes, but a standard-size bagel is actually three to four servings of grains.

# Kara's Weight-Control Plan

I was going to call this my diet plan, but I hate the word *diet*—it's way too loaded with negative connotations. I get asked all the time about what I eat, how much I eat, if I have weight issues—all that stuff. So here's my plan. These principles may not all work for you, but I think they're reasonable. I hope they help.

- **Beware of emotional eating.** Learn to eat only when you are truly physically hungry, and channel negative emotions into things other than eating.
- **Learn to cook** and prepare your own meals as often as possible. It's not that hard!
- **Educate yourself about proper sports nutrition and weight management** by working with a good sports nutritionist or reading a good book on the subject.
- **Don't starve yourself.** Never try to sustain a caloric deficit of more than 200 to 300 calories a day when training and trying to lose weight, and don't skip meals.
- **Eat five to seven times a day** to manage your appetite and keep your metabolism elevated.
- **Include a balance of carbohydrates, healthy fats, and protein** in each meal for lasting energy and appetite control.
- **Weigh yourself consistently (once a day at most!).** This habit keeps you in touch with your goal of getting and staying lean and enables you to respond to weight creep quickly.
- **Include strength training and faster running** in your training program. Both can help make you fitter and leaner.

MAKE GROCERY SHOPPING A PRIORITY SO THAT YOU HAVE PLENTY OF GRAB-AND-GO SNACKS AND FRUIT ON HAND: This is important when you're trying to eat healthfully. Otherwise, at those times when you're hurrying out the door and can't find anything quick, you stop at the doughnut shop on the way to work, or grab something yummy but high-fat from the work refrigerator.

# A Weight-Loss Plan That Works

*Forget the fads and the silly, unrealistic promises. A reasonable weight-loss plan simply has to create a daily calorie deficit. Here's the plan.*

Most women runners will lose body fat by eating between 1,600 and 2,000 calories a day. The following food guide shows you 1,800 calories of healthy, balanced foods. Divide foods into three meals and at least one snack per day.

## What You Can Eat Every Day and Still Lose Weight

3 milk servings

7 grain/starch servings

7 protein equivalents

4 fruit servings

4 vegetable servings (nonstarchy)

4 fat servings

Here are great-tasting food ideas (including appropriate serving size) from each of the preceding six categories:

**Milk/Dairy** (Each serving contains 12 g carbohydrate, 8 g protein.)

- 1 cup skim or 1% milk
- 1 cup nonfat yogurt (120 cal. or less)
- 1 oz. low-fat ice cream or frozen yogurt

**Starches/Grains** (Each serving contains 15 g carbohydrates and 2 g protein.)

- 1 oz. bread or roll (average slice)
- ½ mini bagel, ¼ bagel (4 oz.), 1½ rice cakes
- ½ cup cooked pasta, orzo, polenta, couscous
- ⅓ cup rice, dried beans, low-fat refried beans
- 1 small potato, ½ cup mashed potatoes
- ½ cup starchy vegetable (winter squash, corn, peas)
- ½ English muffin, hamburger or hot dog bun
- ½ cup cooked cereal, ¾ cup dried cereal (1 oz.)

**Protein/Meat and Substitutes** (Each serving contains 7 g protein, 3 g fat.)

- 1 oz. chicken, fish, or lean meat (3 oz. = the size of a deck of cards)
- ¼ cup water-packed tuna
- 1 tbsp. peanut butter
- 1 egg or 2 egg whites
- 1 oz. low-fat cheese (part skim)

**Fruit/Beverage** (Each serving contains 12 g carbohydrates.)

- 1 average-sized piece of fresh fruit
- ½ banana, pear, grapefruit
- 4 oz. juice
- 8 oz. Gatorade
- 2 tbsp. dried fruit

**Vegetables** (Each serving contains 5 g carbohydrates.)

- ½ cup cooked vegetables
- 1 cup raw vegetables
- 1 artichoke
- ½ cup vegetable juice

**Fats/Alcohol** (Each serving contains 5 g fat. *Note:* There's no fat in alcohol.)

- 1 tsp. margarine or butter
- 2 tsp. diet or low-fat margarine
- 1 tbsp. salad dressing, sour cream
- 1 tsp. mayonnaise
- 1 tsp. oil
- 6–8 whole nuts
- ¼ avocado
- 1 slice bacon
- 2 tbsp. lite salad dressing
- 2 tsp. lite mayonnaise
- 1 tbsp. cream cheese

You can substitute one of the following for 2 fats:

- 6 oz. wine
- 1 beer (subtract 1 starch from budget)
- 1 oz. vodka, gin, scotch, bourbon

Putting everything together into a menu, a sample 1,800-calorie day of weight loss may look like this:

## Breakfast

1 cup oatmeal

1 cup nonfat milk

2 tbsp. raisins

1 scrambled egg

## Lunch

turkey wrap on whole wheat tortilla (2 oz. turkey, lettuce, tomato)

small mixed green salad, with 1 tbsp. light vinegrette

1 orange

1 cup strawberry nonfat yogurt

## Afternoon Snack

nonfat latte, 12 oz.

16 almonds

apple

## Dinner

4 oz. flank steak

1 cup brown rice

1 cup steamed asparagus

½ cup berries

6 oz. white wine

**ORGANIZE YOUR FRIDGE AND CUPBOARDS TO MAKE HEALTHY EATING EASY:** First, throw out those tempting refined foods such as cookies, crackers, and potato chips. Then put the healthy stuff front and center in the fridge and in the food cupboards—making it easy to grab. For example, wash the grapes and put them in a bowl on the main shelf in the fridge rather than keeping them in a plastic bag tucked in the back of the bottom bin. Same goes for other fruit. With string cheese, keep the individual pieces front and center in the fridge, not hidden in a bin. As for your cupboards, try making up 100-calorie (give or take!) bags of trail mix using cold cereal, dried nuts, and dried fruit.

**EAT WHEN YOU'RE HUNGRY; STOP WHEN YOU'RE FULL:** Simple as that. No need to wait for your stomach to push against your waistband as your signal to stop.

**HAVE HEALTHY ALTERNATIVES AT THE READY TO DIVERT YOU FROM EMOTIONAL EATING:** A massage or pedicure always works fine, but if you need something more immediate, drinking a tall glass of water may do it. Or make yourself wait 5 minutes before eating and see if the feeling passes (it usually does). Or take a 5-minute walk around the block whether you're at home or at work. When you come back, do a quick reassessment: Am I really hungry?

**THINK OF BREAKING YOUR CALORIES INTO THIRDS:** Eat a third before lunch, another third before dinner, and a third between dinner and evening snacks. Think about eating six smaller meals or three meals and one snack, whichever works best for you.

175

# I LOVE THIS QUOTE

Avoid any diet that discourages the use of hot fudge.
—Don Kardong, marathoner and 1976 U.S. Olympian

I love this quote because it reminds us as runners not to get too caught up in our diets. A little hot fudge every now and then isn't going to kill you. It might make you happier!

# CHAPTER 7

# RACING

What happens when you finally complete (or come close to completing, as it's never truly finished) your running success puzzle? I'll tell you what happened to me. It wasn't quite an overnight success. I suffered an injury soon after I joined the Nike Oregon Project, but once that was behind me, I quickly began to enjoy the benefits of everything I was doing with the team. At the end of the summer 2005 track season, I ran a 5,000m race and set an 11-second personal record (PR), running 15:17. It was my first PR since college, which felt great, but the best thing about it was that I accomplished it with just 45 to 50 miles per week of running. How much faster could I go if I was able to stay healthy and run more? I was about to find out.

At the professional level, the cross-country season falls in the winter. After that promising 5K, I set my sights on the 2006 USA Cross Country Championships in February. A mild achilles tendon injury slowed me down a little and I finished seventh in the 4K race (which is no longer contested), missing out on a qualifying slot for the World Championships in Fukuoka, Japan, by one position. But Lauren Fleshman, who finished ahead of me, was injured eight days before the World Championships and I was sent as her replacement. Even though it took another person's misfortune for me to get that opportunity, it had a powerful effect on my psyche. It was my first chance to represent the United States in international competition and I ran pretty well, finishing as the second American. I realized then that the talent I'd thought I might have lost or maybe never really had was still inside me. My dreams were still alive.

Thankfully, I stayed healthy through the remainder of 2006. As a result, I experienced one of the most enjoyable years of running in my life to that point. I immersed myself in a full European track season, competing in all of the exotic Old World cities I had watched Adam race in five years earlier. I raced with total freedom, choosing a 1,500m one week, a 5,000m the next, open to any possibility in terms of my performance. I set PRs and met the World Championships qualifying standards at every distance, finishing the year ranked number two in the United States at 3,000m and 5,000m and number one at 10,000m.

In the winter I took some time off from training not because an injury forced me to but simply to refresh myself. A novelty. When I returned to training in early 2007, I was ready to take my running to the next level. As I've mentioned, putting the puzzle together is partly about figuring out what works best for you and what doesn't work and adapting your training accordingly. In our first two-plus years of working together, Alberto and I learned a lot about my individual training needs. Our plan for 2007 was to race sparingly and commit ourselves to the training formula that seemed right for me. One thing we learned was that I could handle a heavy load of hard running when healthy, so we heaped it on like never before. I started running my first 80-mile weeks, and my body liked them.

In the summer I qualified for the World Championships in Osaka, Japan, by finishing second at the U.S. Championships behind Deena Kastor in the 10,000m. When we returned home to Portland from In-dianapolis, where the championships were held, Alberto told me to do whatever I wanted for a week. "And then I'm going to train you harder than you've ever trained in your life," he said.

On Saturday, June 30, early in that week off, I decided to go for an easy run around the Nike campus. While I was running, I saw an ambulance with flashing lights drive onto the campus. As I finished the run, at the field house I saw the ambulance leaving in a hurry. I walked toward the front door and saw Galen Rupp, Josh Rohatinsky (another runner on our team), and Josh's brother Jared standing outside. Something about the scene looked odd.

"Hi guys," I said. "How's it going?" Then I noticed that Galen's face looked as if all the blood had been drained out of it.

"Alberto just had a heart attack," he said.

I won't describe the scramble of the next few hours and days. I will only say that Alberto pulled through, thank heavens. And not only that, but he did not even change the plans he had made to take Galen, Adam, and me to a high-altitude training camp in Park City, Utah. That camp probably would have been a bonding experience for the four of us anyway, but given what we had just gone through, it brought us even closer together.

It also did something very special for my running. I was on an upswing already, but almost losing Alberto changed my perspective on my career and life. I felt the preciousness of every opportunity as I never had before. My last few key workouts in August before flying to Japan were some of the best I'd ever done. Alberto, who always sets high expectations but never encourages unrealistic goals, began to speak to me seriously about the possibility of a medal.

"You can do this," he told me when it came time to make a race plan. "Don't think. Just stay glued to whoever's in front. When they go, you go. I'd rather see you blow up trying to win and finish tenth than run conservatively and finish fourth."

I halfway believed in Alberto's belief and halfway doubted him. I showed my doubt when I tried to leave my hotel in Osaka without my

179

RACING

medal ceremony warm-up suit, which I would need to wear if I finished in the top three. Adam protested.

"You're going to need it," he said.

"No, I'm not. Besides, there's no room in my bag."

"Then I'll take it," he said, stuffing the suit in his own bag. Given what happened later that evening, this story would be better if the medal ceremony had taken place immediately after the race, as we assumed it would. Instead, it was scheduled for the next day. So I did not, in fact, need the warm-ups—but not for the reason I thought!

While my confidence did not match Alberto's and Adam's, my desire did, and I stuck to the plan. I did not think. I just ran. It was a hot night and the race started slowly, as championship distance events often do. At the end of the twentieth lap, with five laps to go, I was in second place. But then the defending world champion, Tirunesh Dibaba of Ethiopia, threw down an aggressive surge that caught me off guard and suddenly I was behind six other girls. I gathered my wits and chased the leaders, clawing my way back into third place over the next lap and a half. By this point, I was suffering badly, and when Joanne Pavey of Great Britain passed me with 800 meters left in the race, I thought it was all over—for a moment.

Then I thought about all the work I had done to get here. I recalled running while wearing a garbage bag to prepare for the heat that was now boiling my muscles. All I had to do to validate all of that work was to bear the pain another minute or so. With 200 meters to go, Jo was still within reach in front of me. *I have to go now!* I thought. I got up on my toes, drove my arms, and sprinted with all the life inside me. I pulled even with Jo's shoulder and dragged myself ahead. *Please, let this crush her will!* I thought. When I hit the finish line, I was still in third place. I had won a World Championship bronze medal! I couldn't believe it.

That moment was life-changing in the most basic sense. Suddenly the girl who had to sell herself to college coaches and later to shoe companies was sought after. Immediately after my triumph in Osaka, the organizers of the Great North Run, a major half marathon in New-castle, England, offered me a large appearance fee to square off against Paula Radcliffe, the world's greatest female distance runner.

# CAN'T-MISS TIPS FOR EVERY RACE, WHETHER IT'S YOUR FIRST RACE OR YOUR ONE HUNDREDTH

E ven if you're not into racing, promise me that you'll at least read the advice in this chapter. I feel confident that once you do, you'll be ready to give racing a try.

The way I see it—and race veterans will back me up on this—races encapsulate the best aspects of our sport, which can make races incredibly moving experiences. The camaraderie. The emotion. The wonderful variety of body shapes and sizes. The challenge of something pure. The simplicity of the task. The inclusiveness you feel among participants. The respect shown for speedsters and slowpokes alike. For the price you pay to enter a road race, you really get a lot out of it!

Of course, racing also involves anxiety. Doubt. Even fear. But that's all part of the attraction. Meaningful ventures always come with these feelings. I'll be the first to tell you that I've been a basket case before some of my races—so much so that I could hardly talk. But this just makes it even sweeter when you meet the challenge once that starting gun goes off, and conquer it. There are few better things in this world than the feeling you get after a race well run—whether that means winning it or finishing it.

These tips will help you in your next race—guaranteed.

**BE OKAY WITH THAT "SLUGGO" FEELING THE WEEK PRECEDING YOUR RACE:** This is natural, so just relax and tell yourself you have done the training and you will feel great on race morning. Sometimes it's just nerves that are causing the feeling; sometimes it's your body adjusting to running fewer miles than during your race buildup. Sometimes it's both—hate that! I've found that it sometimes helps to go for a short run—just 2 to 3 miles—during which you throw in some short speed surges. This can snap you out of your funk.

**BE OKAY WITH THAT FEELING OF "I'M GETTING SICK—I JUST KNOW IT:"** For some runners, the days before the big race are all about the blahs (see previous tip). For others in those final days, it's the mysterious illness that comes on, threatening to ruin everything. I shouldn't joke because I know this can be awful, but ninety-nine times out of a hundred, this "sickness" is just nerves manifesting themselves in a really annoying way. So be determined to ignore it or laugh it off. If by chance you are coming down with something, you'll know it on race day and can make adjustments accordingly.

**STAY OFF YOUR FEET THE DAY BEFORE (BUT NO NEED TO BE OBSESSIVE ABOUT IT):** If you have traveled to a race, the temptation will be to do some touring, especially if your family or a friend is with you. Fight that temptation. Or take a guided bus tour instead, or a ferryboat tour. Some walking is completely fine—you're fit, after all—but keep it moderate. Watching an inspirational movie the night before is always a good option.

**BE ORGANIZED ON RACE MORNING:** Arriving late and frazzled is no way to show up at a race. To be sure you show up primed and ready, remember the following:

- Set out all your racing clothes and gear the night before so that you know exactly where everything is when you get up.

# DEAR KARA

**You always used to hear that having sex the night before a race would hurt your performance, and I actually believe it. My husband thinks I'm being ridiculous about this. Should I stick with my habit or, um, get with his program?**

Without giving you too much information on my own life, I personally haven't seen a difference either way. I think that you should pick a race that isn't that important to you and give your husband's program a try. You could even do it before a hard workout if you are too nervous to risk a race. What's the worst that happens? If you have a bad day, big deal. But if you have a great day, you'll be happy you tried and so will your husband!

- Wake up in plenty of time and have a light bite to eat.
- Arrive at the race early, with enough time to visit the bathroom, then do an easy jog warm-up, a few quick strides, and a light stretch.
- Find a quiet spot and take 2 or 3 minutes to visualize the success you will have that day.
- Make your way to the start, and keep walking or jogging in place until the gun sounds so that you keep your heart rate up and muscles loose.

**PUT ON SOME EXTRA DEODORANT:** Yes, you might be racing with a bunch of men, but there's no reason to smell like one.

**GET YOUR HAIR FIGURED OUT:** Wearing it down on a training run is one thing—there's no pressure to perform on those days. But in a race, you'll want everything just so in order to concentrate on the task at hand. So put your hair up or back and make sure it's secure (you don't want to fuss with it while you're racing).

**TAKE CARE OF AREAS THAT MIGHT CHAFE.** This is especially key for longer races, but skin chafing and blisters can happen in 5Ks and 10Ks as well, especially if it's raining (blisters love the rain). Problem areas include the nipples, along bra lines, under the arms, and between the thighs. Before the race starts, use either Vaseline to guard against chafing or specialized skin lube that's made for runners, which tends not to stain or be as messy as Vaseline. Two other strategies that can help:

- Wear high-tech fabrics that wick moisture away from the skin and that dry more quickly.
- Wear broken-in race clothing that you know will work well.

**HAVE AT LEAST TWO GOALS GOING INTO EVERY RACE TO GUARANTEE SUCCESS:** One should be a "stretch" goal, one that challenges you, such as running a certain time, winning an age-group prize, or finishing without walking. The other should be a goal that is very reachable, and it may not be competitive, per se. Examples of these doable but nevertheless important race goals:

- Strike up a conversation with at least one person during the race.
- Feel proud of yourself for getting out there in the first place.
- Work out a recent problem that's been concerning you, either from work or in your private life.
- Dedicate your race to a troubled, sick, or deceased friend or loved one.
- High-five twenty spectators along the route (and be sure five of them are children).
- Give thanks at the finish line that you are healthy and able to run.
- Be completely positive about your performance, regardless of where you placed or how fast you ended up running.

**DRIVE THE COURSE BEFOREHAND:** If you're serious about an upcoming race and are determined to do well, drive the course first. Pay attention to hills, turns, mile marks, and road surface. All the while, try to be constructing a game plan for the race, then visualize that game plan in the days beforehand. Do one last visualization a few minutes before the start.

**DON'T WORRY ABOUT LACK OF SLEEP THE NIGHT BEFORE:** You know how it can be if you have ever done a road race: Tossing. Turning. Should've trained more. Should've trained less. I feel stuffed up—am I getting a cold? It can be pretty awful. I've been there plenty of times. But one thing you don't have to worry about is lack of sleep hurting your performance the next day. It won't. Fortunately, the body doesn't work like that. As long as you've had some decent sleep two and three nights before the race, you'll be absolutely fine.

**KEEP A SPECIAL PAIR OF "SPEED SHOES" FOR RACING ONLY:** You need plenty of cushioning and support in your regular training shoes, but for racing shoes, you may be able to get away with something lighter and sleeker—maybe even flashier. There's a running shoe category called lightweight trainers that might work perfectly for you. Ask about them at the local running store. With half marathons and marathons, you should probably stick with regular training shoes for the long-haul support, but even then, keep a special pair aside for races only. They'll be your secret weapon.

**KEEP A FOR-RACES-ONLY OUTFIT AT THE READY:** Assemble an outfit that you look and feel great in. Perhaps it's a little skimpier than your normal training gear. Maybe it fits a little bit tighter. Maybe the color is a bit louder. And think hat and running shades right down to your socks and running shoes—a complete outfit only for racing.

**STOP DRINKING FLUIDS AT LEAST AN HOUR BEFORE BEDTIME THE NIGHT BEFORE YOUR RACE:** Hydrating is good the day before your race, but that night stop doing it early enough so that you won't have to visit the bathroom multiple times in the middle of the night. It can be tough to get back to sleep afterward.

**REVEL IN YOUR PRERACE ANXIETY:** Admittedly, battling your nerves and doubts before a big race is not always the most fun thing in the world. (Believe me, I've been there.) And when it affects your sleep? Yuck. But in a way this is such a great thing, because it is a sign that the

# IT WORKS FOR ME

**I think it is important to visualize your race with everything going wrong.** We all want to imagine the perfect race, but in reality that is very rare. It's good to imagine yourself working through pain and unexpected obstacles.

**I always take an extra thin pair of socks on race day.** When I change from my trainers to my racing flats, I switch into my new socks. I think having my feet dry at the start helps prevent blisters.

**About a week before a big race, I start making sure I am awake at the time that the race is going to be run.** If it's a late-night race, I try to start sleeping a bit later so that I can be awake later in the day. If it's a morning start, especially if it's in another time zone, I start getting up 30 minutes earlier each day so that it won't be such a shock to my system on race day.

**I always have a thin pair of stretchy gloves that I don't mind losing in my racing bag.** I buy the cheap ones. You never know when it might feel a tad chilly on the start line or in the early part of a race in the late evening or early morning. Once I get going and warm up a bit, I just toss them off.

**If I'm running in a road race and it looks as if the weather is going to be cold, I make sure to wear an old long sleeve top to the start line.** That way I won't get too cold waiting for the race to start and I can throw it off anywhere and not worry about getting it back later.

race really means something to you. How many other things in your life have this effect? Probably not that many. So embrace the feeling; it's part of being a runner who races. And it makes finishing feel that much more fantastic.

**GIVE YOURSELF PLENTY OF TIME FOR THE PORTABLE TOILET:** It can be a very unpleasant feeling indeed to hear the race announcer saying, "5 minutes to the start, everyone move toward the starting line *please!*"—and you're in the back of a long Porta-Potty line that hasn't moved since you arrived. And you really have to go. Number 2. So get to the start early. When you're deciding which Porta-Potty line to get into, look for the one with a high percentage of guys. Men tend to be quicker.

**BE PREPARED TO "SQUAT" IF YOU HAVE TO:** Um, maybe not if we're talking number 2 (sorry, gross!), but my point here is, if you run out of time and the bathroom lines are not moving, you may have to find a discreet spot in the woods. This might sound awful, but you know what? It's a runner thing, and you will very likely have company in there when you do your thing. So don't worry about it—nobody cares. Just get it over with and get back to the race.

**REMEMBER TO WEAR SUNSCREEN, A HAT, AND SHADES:** Especially if you're running a 10K or longer. I can't tell you the number of times I've seen runners finish races with burned foreheads, arms, and shoulders. Plus, running in the bright sunshine without sunglasses will cause you to squint, and squinting will make your face tighten, which can make your neck and shoulders tighten, and so on. Be good to yourself. Stay protected.

**LINE UP IN THE APPROPRIATE AREA AT THE START:** If you're a slow runner, you'll want to get near the back of the crowd lining up at the start. If you're fast, get closer to the banner. Many races have signs posted that

## DEAR KARA

**I wish there were more women-only races, because I can't stand finishing so far back in the pack. What's your opinion on this?**

Don't worry about where you finish in the pack! When there are more people in the race, you have more people for setting your pace. Run your own race and set goals that are right for you. Then you won't worry about something you can't control, like where you finish in the pack.

show minutes-per-mile paces, so just go to the section with your estimated mile pace.

**DON'T BE TIMID ABOUT IT!** Some racing mistakes are made before the gun goes off, and placing yourself in the wrong area of the start is one of those things, especially for women. If you're ready to break 20 minutes for the 5K or something speedy like that, don't let the "boys" shoulder you back to row 20.

**HAVE A PLAN FOR HOW YOU'RE GOING TO RUN THE RACE, BUT HAVE A PLAN B (AND SOMETIMES C) AS WELL:** Your plan doesn't have to be anything elaborate, but you should have it thought out before you start your race. These sorts of examples would work: "I'm going to go out real easy for the first 3 miles. Then, depending on how I feel, I'll try to pick it up (if I'm feeling good) a little in miles 4 and 5, and finish strong over the last mile." Or: "I will do my best to run a 9-minute-mile pace the whole way, like clockwork. If it gets hot or it's just not my day, I'll back off to 9:30 miles. If I'm feeling great at halfway, I'll pick it up to 8:45 miles and try to hold that pace the rest of the way."

**BE PATIENT WHEN THE STARTING GUN SOUNDS—SOMETIMES YOU DON'T MOVE FOR SEVERAL MINUTES:** Especially if you're a slower runner at a large race, literally thousands of runners will cross the starting line in front of you, so it can take some time before you get moving. Just jog in place, shuffle along, and soon enough you'll be running free. And it's not as if you're losing time or falling off your pace. Your official time doesn't start until you cross the starting line.

**FOCUS ON YOURSELF DURING A RACE, NOT SO MUCH ON THOSE AROUND YOU:** If you think about others, invariably you'll be hit with thoughts like: "She looks faster than me." Or: "She's not even sweating." Or: "I'm breathing so much harder than she is. What's wrong?" Keep things inner directed. Be aware of others, but keep yourself front and center.

# I LOVE THIS QUOTE

Every athlete has doubts. Elite runners in particular are insecure people. You need someone to affirm that what you are doing is right.

—Lynn Jennings

I love this quote because even though a lot of runners don't want to admit it, we all have our doubts. You absolutely need to have a person you trust who can assure you that you are on the right path.

**TAKE THE FIRST FEW TURNS *WIDE*:** If there are tight turns early in a big road race, approach them a bit wider rather than "running the tangents," as we say in running. This way you'll avoid the traffic jam effect—runners piling up on the inside of a turn in an effort to run the shortest distance between two points.

191

**LINE UP ON THE OPPOSITE SIDE OF THE FIRST TURN:** Continuing with the theme of the preceding tip, some races with mass starts include a big

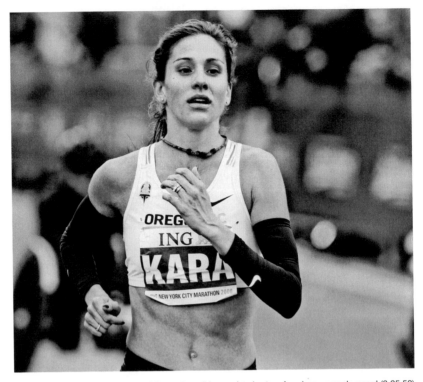

**A QUICK STUDY:** Thanks to smart training and a solid race plan, I set an American women's record (2:25:53) for a debut marathon at New York in 2008.

turn that comes early on, within the first half mile. If that's the case and you can see the turn, line up at the start on the *opposite* side of that turn (i.e., if the turn goes left, line up on the right) so that you don't get "pinched" in the bottleneck of runners heading straight for the turn.

**THINK EVEN *EFFORT,* NOT EVEN PACE:** You always hear that the key to successful racing is running at an even pace throughout (at least until your Olympic-style sprint at the end!). In a road race with hills, however, that's not the smartest method. The key is to run even effort, which means slowing up a little on the uphills (when gravity is working against you) and speeding up a little on the downhills (when gravity is working for you). By the end of the race, the net outcome will be an evenly paced race, but the efficient manner in which you got there will be the key.

## DEAR KARA

**I'm a very competitive person and sometimes it bugs me that some men are faster than me just because they're men and have stronger, bigger muscles. Does this ever bother you?**

It used to bother me that I am a world-class female athlete and a pretty good high school boy could beat me. But at this point I've accepted it and moved on. There is nothing you can do about it. Just be the best you can be and don't obsess over the fact that men are faster than women. That's life.

**PASS RUNNERS WITH AUTHORITY:** If you're the competitive type and race frequently, this tip is for you. When you're coming up on a fellow racer fairly slowly and are about to pass him or her, put on just a little burst of speed as you go by. Keep it up until you're well past—maybe 20 to 30 yards in front of that person—then slip back to your normal pace. Otherwise, I've found from experience that the runner you're passing will often "latch on" as you go by, because they think it will help them stay with the pace. But, if you go by him with authority, he won't even try to stay with you, as clearly you're out of his league.

**BREAK THE RACE INTO SEGMENTS:** Depending on how long the race is, it's good mental strategy to divide it into segments so that it's not so daunting. It's like with any task, really. You take care of this part, then this part, then this part, and suddenly you've finished the job. With a 5K it's probably not as necessary, but even here it'll help to think mile 1, mile 2, then mile 3. What's more, the trick is to think about these sections individually and customize your strategy to each. For example, experienced half marathoners often divide that race into

193

the first 5 miles, the second 5 miles, and the final 3.1 miles. Many will often have a different plan for each section, such as go supereasy for the first 5, concentrate on pace for the second 5, and push hard for the final 3.1. Try it out in your next race, and be sure to have your framework figured out before the start.

**BE PREPARED FOR THE INEVITABLE "BAD PATCH":** Runners in the United Kingdom coined the term "bad patch" to relate to racing, and it has to do with those times in a race when you either lose concentration or suddenly feel down mentally, or otherwise simply lose the plot. In a long race especially, this can be very disconcerting, because rationally you know you should be fine, but emotionally you can start to panic with thoughts of "Oh no, what's going on—am I going to have to quit?" No, you won't have to quit; you just have to weather the bad patch. Normally it passes within a minute or two. One way to get through it is simply to latch on to a runner or runners nearby and let them pace you along until you get yourself back together. Another method is to let yourself slow down ever so slightly, as a way of "letting yourself off the hook" until you recover your momentum.

# I LOVE THIS QUOTE

Running is a lot like life. Only 10 percent of it is exciting;
90 percent of it is slog and drudge.
—Dave Bedford, English distance runner who
occasionally puts in 200 miles a week in training

I love this quote because this is the essence of training for competition. Most of the time, you are in pain, pushing your body and mind through workouts and runs. But every once in a while, you have that one race or one training session that is magical and that keeps you fighting through the misery for more. You continue on, just hoping for a taste of the magic again.

**THANK THE RACE VOLUNTEERS AS YOU PASS THEM:** Volunteering for a race certainly has its fun and inspiring moments—and I recommend you try it if you haven't yet—but it certainly has an unsung hero aspect to it as well. For example, aid station volunteers often arrive long before the race to set things up, then they're handing out drinks and picking up empty cups during the race, then they have to clean everything up afterward. Not exactly glamorous work. So yell a word of thanks or encouragement as you're running by. They'll appreciate it a lot.

**WHEN APPROACHING AID STATIONS OR WATER STOPS, GO TO THE FAR END FOR YOUR DRINK:** It happens every time at big and even small races. People clamor for water or a sport drink at the first part of the first table they come to, and suddenly there's a traffic jam of runners reaching over, under, and around their fellow runners trying to grab their drinks. Play it smart and keep running beyond this congestion point, aiming for a section a little farther along. Voilà, smooth drink delivery.

**MAKE EYE CONTACT AND SIGNAL YOUR INTENT TO GRAB:** More good water stop strategy here. It can be confusing and a bit frantic at these places, so as you approach a volunteer who is holding out a cup, look her in the eye and point to the cup she's holding for you so that she knows your intent.

**REMEMBER TO PINCH THE CUP:** An old trick that works well for drinking at water stops is to pinch the top of the cup to narrow the opening you drink through. This creates a funnel, which will better direct the fluid into your mouth rather than all over the front of your T-shirt. Oh, and when you're done drinking, toss the cup way off to the side of the road

195

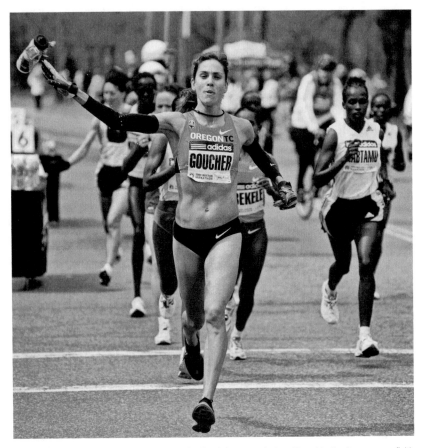

**FLUID DYNAMICS:** Elite runners grab their own bottles during races, but you'll want to develop your own fluid-station techniques to help you stay well hydrated.

so that other runners won't step on it. Unless there's a bin to toss it into, in which case use that.

**SEE OTHER RACERS AS "POSITIVE PROPS":** Use your fellow competitors as positive energy sources to help you in your quest to run your best, as opposed to seeing them as negative obstacles who are working against you. You're all competing together.

**RUN NEXT TO PEOPLE, NOT RIGHT BEHIND THEM:** Sometimes it's tempting to tuck in behind other runners, perhaps to get a break from the wind, or because you find a runner who looks strong and you want to stay with that person for a while. But it's not fair to do this for long (a few seconds is fine), and it's annoying to the person in front of you. Better to come up beside that person and both work together.

**TAKE A TURN AT THE FRONT IF YOU'RE IN A PROTECTIVE PACK:** In windy conditions, it's natural for packs of runners to form as a break against the wind. If you find yourself in one, it's considered proper running etiquette to do some time at the front, to help break the wind for others. That said, once you're in the late stages of the race—the last mile or so—it is every racer for herself!

**SOAK IN THE ENERGY; REVEL IN THE APPLAUSE:** There is a ton of energy at road races that comes from both the runners and the spectators. Make the most of that—take it on board and store it for when you need it later in the race. And people clapping for you? You can't beat that! How often does that happen to you at work when you're putting yourself out there and trying your best?

## I LOVE THIS QUOTE

Everyone in life is looking for a certain rush. Racing is where I get mine.

—John Trautmann, former round and track star

I love this quote because it describes me. Nothing thrills me more than lining up on a starting line getting ready to see if I can pull off a big feat. Racing is the greatest thrill of my life.

**WRITE YOUR NAME ON YOUR TOP:** Many races have started printing first names in big letters on the race numbers you wear on the front of your torso. Great idea. It is so motivating to have hundreds and sometimes thousands of spectators yelling your name during the course of a race. This happened to me at the New York City Marathon a couple of years ago and it was amazing. But if you run a race that doesn't do this, write your name in big letters on the front of one of your race T-shirts. Some runners even write things like "Go, Gail, Go!" which works nicely as well.

**GET FASTER EACH MILE:** It would be tough to play this pacing game in a marathon, but in your next shorter race, try to go faster with each mile. It will mean starting out very conservatively, but that's a good thing to do anyway. Gradually increase your speed until you are really moving out over the last mile. This is an exhilarating way to race, and you'll feel great after your fast finish.

**BREATHE FROM WAY DOWN IN THE BELLY:** This will take practice, but it works best to do "belly breathing" when you train and race. This ensures you get a big, deep breath and aren't doing that almost hyperventilating style of shallow breathing that too many runners do.

**BREATHE NORMALLY—AND THROUGH THE MOUTH!** You occasionally still hear the old running wive's tale (husband's tale?) about needing to breathe through the nose when you run, as this warms the air on cold days or otherwise does a better job of filtering. Not so! Just breathe the way you always do, which is normally through the mouth.

**GO BY FEEL, NOT BY THE CLOCK:** At plenty of races it's tough to get away from the clock, as you get your split times every mile on big digital devices that are impossible to miss. But every once in a while, go to a race with the idea that you're not going to wear a watch or pay any attention to the mile-split clocks. Instead, run naturally. Set a pace that feels right, then just take the race as it comes. Slow down on the uphills, speed up on the downhills, go a little faster when you're feeling good, slow down when you're feeling fatigued, and so on. You might be surprised how liberating this feels.

**SHIFT INTO "CLIMBING GEAR" ON STEEP UPHILLS:** I've found that it really works to visualize this downshifting phenomenon, like you do in a standard transmission car, or when you put a mountain bike in first gear and can climb just about anything. That's what you want to think about when you come to a big hill in a race. Really shorten your running stride as well so that you baby-step your way to the top (trying to "eat up" ground with big strides absolutely does not work going uphill). Keep your head up as well, and look toward the top of the hill. This will keep you from hunching forward into the hill, which is much less efficient.

**GET ACTIVE WITH YOUR ARMS:** Like a lot of these race tips, this advice works for your regular training runs; it's just that much more critical in a race. A more active arm swing and a slightly exaggerated, "snappy" knee lift will help propel you up big hills. On steep descents, try lowering your arms a little bit and holding them slightly wider to provide better stability.

**THEN "FLOAT" DOWN THE OTHER SIDE:** This goes for regular training runs, too, of course, but in a race where you're expending more effort, it's key to run lightly on your feet going downhill. Pretend you're running on eggshells that you don't want to break. If you're pounding with each step, that's inefficient, and it's going to needlessly slow you down. Plus there's a good chance it's going to make you more sore after the race.

**MAKE TIME ON THE DOWNHILLS:** If you're looking to carve 15 to 20 seconds off your personal best—and those seconds have been frustratingly elusive—try putting a little more effort into your downhills. That's right, downhills, *not* uphills. A lot of recreational racers think that to go faster they need to charge up hills, but they fail to take advantage of the downhills. That's a missed opportunity. So again, drop your arms slightly, hold them out away from your body somewhat for more stability, then lean with the hill a little bit, like a skier. This will boost your speed without you spending any extra energy, and it will translate to several seconds over the course of a hilly race.

**CONTINUE TO "GLIDE" AT THE BOTTOM:** This old trick is from running expert and former Olympian Jeff Galloway. The idea is to extend your downhill speed to the flat part at the bottom of the hill, thereby taking advantage of your gravity-induced momentum for several more seconds. This makes for a more fluid, efficient effort as you descend from each hill.

**APPRECIATE RACING FOR THE HONEST TEST THAT IT IS:** To quote Oprah Winfrey: "Running is the greatest metaphor for life, because you get out of it what you put into it." Racing may be even more like that. You run from point A to point B and get timed for it. No machines to help get you there, no assistance from team members, no help from technology (okay, your shoes help a little bit). Very few endeavors in life allow for such honest, unfiltered feedback on your effort.

**BE CONSERVATIVE EARLY, BOLD LATER ON:** On very hilly courses especially, consider a strategy of gradual aggression; that is, avoid the temptation to "push" the first few hills, and instead save something for the latter ones—especially in a long race, or a race where the big hills loom later in the route.

# I LOVE THIS QUOTE

Racing teaches us to challenge ourselves. It teaches us to push
beyond where we thought we could go. It helps us to find out what
we are made of. This is what we do. This is what it's all about.
—PattiSue Plumer, U.S. Olympian

I love this quote because I love what PattiSue is saying. My favorite
thing about running is racing. I love the challenge. I love discovering
how much more I can get out of my body. Until you try, you never know.

**BE READY TO ANSWER THE QUESTION:** Anyone who has ever run to their
very limit in a race has faced this phenomenon. It's that point in
the race—and unfortunately sometimes there are several!—when
your body and mind are both asking: Are you going to hang in there
through this pain, or are you going to slow down just a little bit? Tough
question! And you will know exactly how you answered it when you
reach the finish line.

**STOP AND GIVE ASSISTANCE IF NEEDED:** If race volunteers or medical people
are already attending to a fellow competitor during a race, there's no
need to stop. But if someone falls or collapses or looks in distress, stop
to see if you can help. Doing so could save that person's life.

**WEAR YOUR ID IN RACES, TOO:** You already knew it was important to do
this on your training runs, but it is the same with races. If you get into
trouble, it will help those who assist you to know your name, address,
and any pertinent medical conditions you may have. Also, be sure you
tell your estimated finishing time to anyone who comes to cheer you
on so that they can alert race officials if you don't show up.

**RACE THE CONDITIONS:** You've trained for months for a particular race
and everything has gone perfectly. But race day arrives, you head to

the starting line, and it's 95 degrees with high humidity. What do you do? *Take it slow and easy.* There's absolutely no fighting that kind of heat. Same goes for high wind, rain, bitter cold, or even a course that's way hillier than you expected. Be realistic. Be smart.

## ON THE CONTRARY

**I don't visualize winning the race or thinking ahead to the finish when I'm racing.** It makes me do silly things and veer from my plan. I try to stay only in the moment that I'm in and focus on what I should be doing at that exact moment in the race.

**I know a lot of people worry about getting a good sleep the night before a race, but I really focus on resting two to three nights out.** The night before, my head is racing and sleep doesn't always come easy. If I've slept well the two nights before, I know I'm plenty rested, so I don't worry about the night before.

**RUN TALL AND SMILE BIG WHEN YOU PASS THE RACE PHOTOGRAPHER:** Sometimes in a race, you don't see the photographer until it's too late. Result: grim face, staring at feet, furrowed brow. So keep an eye out and be ready to look your best when you run by.

**CONSIDER BUILDING IN REGULAR WALK BREAKS:** This tip would've caused gasping and vigorous head-shaking among runners a few years ago, but now it's just considered smart strategy in long races such as marathons. The walking will extend your endurance and keep you fresher longer. The key is to do the walk breaks from the beginning of the race; don't wait until you have to walk because you're exhausted. As such, this is a proactive, not a reactive race strategy. You have some options:

- Walk through every aid station, which helps you drink properly as well.
- Walk a minute at every mile stop.

- Walk for 2 minutes every 2 miles.
- Run 5 miles, walk 1 mile, run 5 miles, and so on.

**LOOK INTO A CORPORATE CHALLENGE RACE AND ENTER A TEAM OF YOUR CO-WORKERS:** The JP Morgan Chase Corporate Challenge is the biggest of these sorts of events (it's worldwide), but there are many others besides. They're quite fun and informal. You get a bunch of your work-mates to sign up, everyone trains for the race, then you run it together and are scored as a team. Race distances are quite manageable—usually 3 or 3.5 miles. A really nice spinoff possibility is that upper management looks very favorably on these efforts (major brownie points for you), and oftentimes the increased corporate fitness aware-ness among employees leads to an upgrade of on-site workout facilities, on-site employee health fairs and health screenings, and corporate discounts to nearby gyms and nutrition stores.

## DEAR KARA

**I've been a runner for almost five years, but I have never run a race. I'm a little intimidated by it. Can you help?**
Your first race can be a very intimidating experience. You don't have to race to be a runner. But if it is something that you want to do, you should go for it. Ask a friend or a relative to do the race with you. Then you can get through your first one without feeling alone. Once you have accomplished your first race, the next one won't feel so scary. Good luck!

203

**SOAK UP THE ENERGY FROM THE BANDS AT RACES, BUT DON'T GET CARRIED AWAY:** Lots of big half marathons and marathons have bands along the way, and they can really perk you up when you run by. Sometimes it's tempting to just stop and listen to the music instead! Just be careful, as music can sometimes inspire you to go faster than you should—like up that steep hill at mile 5 of the Heavy Metal 10K. Keep your pace under control, and store the energy the music provides. You may need it later.

**COUNT STEPS IF THINGS GET TOUGH:** This tip relates a little to the "bad patch" tip. Sometimes if you hit a point in the race where you're really struggling, it's best to try to shut off the negative chatter your brain is starting to fixate on. One way is to start counting your steps. That's it—just start counting. When you get to 100, start over at 1. This can take your mind off your troubles and get you back on track.

**COUNT *DOWN* THE MILES, NOT UP, AS YOU NEAR THE FINISH:** In a marathon, for example, the race always provides mile marks that count up to 26. But once you start hitting 16, then 17, then 18, then later 22 and 23, that can start to seem like a really big number. As in, am I actually running that far? A better psychological ploy is—once you reach mile 15 or so in a marathon, or mile 8 or 9 in a half marathon—to start counting down. So at mile 16 you say, "10 to go"; at mile 17 you say, "9 to go"; and so on. The numbers start getting smaller and smaller, which is a whole lot nicer for your brain to process than larger and larger numbers.

**SPREAD YOUR SUPPORT CREW AROUND THE COURSE:** Whatever the distance you run, it's awfully nice to have family and friends come cheer for you. Make the most of this by getting them to fan out so that you see them at different points on the course. Maybe they can ride bicycles to make this easier. See if they can station themselves halfway up tough hills, or at turnaround points or at particularly lonely spots on the course.

**IGNORE THE SILLY GUY STUFF:** Some men will break into a sprint if a woman pulls up on their shoulder during a race. Let them. Just hold your pace. When you catch this person the second or third time, let him do it again. Then counterattack with everything you have as you approach the finish.

## DEAR KARA

**In lots of the races I run, the prize money for men is more than it is for women. I don't like that. Does this bother you, too?**
As a self-proclaimed feminist, this bothers me a lot. I am also irritated by coverage given to men versus women on television, newspapers, magazines, and so on. But at the end of the day, I am running for myself and the joy it has brought to my life. I'm not going to let the irritation I feel when I see discrimination take away the joy I get from running.

**PAY FOR EVERY RACE IN WHICH YOU PARTICIPATE:** People who run races without officially entering them are called bandits. Don't be a bandit. Bandits take advantage of race resources without doing their part to pay for them. Some bandits do even worse things, like pretend to complete a race when in fact they cut part of the course. Electronic timing chips have made this more difficult to do, but it still happens. Report banditry when you see it!

**KICK FROM FARTHER OUT:** Strong, spirited finishing kicks are not just for the elite runners. It's always great to pick it up at the end. But no need for last-10-seconds, head-back sprinting, either. Rather, aim for a longer, smoother, well-paced kick from 90 seconds or even 2 minutes out from the finish line. Don't wait (like many do) for merely the last 100 meters when the finish line actually appears.

**FEAR NOT IF YOU ARE LAST:** Coming in last is probably the most common fear that people have about entering their first race. Given that there are so many walkers in road races these days, it is extremely unlikely that you'll come in last as long as you run for at least a few minutes of the race. If you do come in last, just ahead of the "sweeper" ambulance, so what? You'll get a bigger ovation than anyone except the winners. And sometimes bigger than them.

**CONGRATULATE THE RUNNERS THAT FINISH WITH YOU:** Chances are good that you were running with some of these people for a mile or two or even more at the end of the race. But regardless, you finished at the same time, and it's nice to acknowledge that with a "good going" or a "well done" when you're finally across the finish line. A quick hug works well sometimes!

**TAKE A FEW MINUTES TO CHEER FOR OTHERS COMING IN AFTER YOU FINISH:** You'll probably want to get your medal, a drink, and a bagel or banana first, but then loop back around to the finish area if it's accessible and cheer for runners coming in after you. They'll appreciate it, and it's inspiring for you as well.

**STICK AROUND FOR THE AWARDS CEREMONY:** Even if you're not expecting to win any awards, it's good sportsmanship to be there to clap for those who do win them. I've been to races in the past where the weather is bad or it's really cold, and the crowds have pretty much all gone home by the time the awards ceremony happens. Those are the times when it's even more important to stick around.

**WEAR YOUR RACE MEDAL PROUDLY THE EVENING AFTER THE RACE:** I love this custom among runners. Especially at really big races, it's so cool to see so many runners on the streets and in restaurants and bars wearing their medals with pride. You deserve it, so do it! It's kind of funny, though, as you can usually tell who the runners are anyway, regardless of the medals around their necks. They look tired but happy and relieved, and they're usually walking quite slowly and deliberately from leg soreness!

**EAT AND DRINK WHATEVER YOU WANT:** I mean this within reason, of course, especially regarding alcohol. But seriously, if there was ever a time when you deserved a guilt-free meal of anything your hungry little heart desires, it's after a good race effort. In practical calorie-burning terms, if you ran a half marathon, you burned an extra 1,300 calories. A marathon? That's 2,600 extra calories. Can you say three scoops of ice cream?

**CONSIDER SENDING A THANK-YOU NOTE THAT INCLUDES SOME SUGGESTIONS:** Race directors love to hear from runners after the race. This doesn't happen very often, which is a shame, because race directors are always

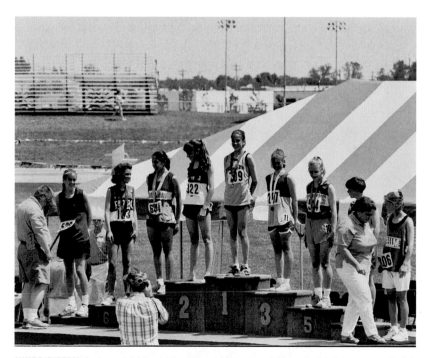

**AWARD SYSTEM:** Saving your finish medals and keeping them in a visible spot will help keep you motivated. Here I (#709) beam with pride thanks to a first-place finish in high school.

trying to make improvements to their events. After your races, send a quick note and mention anything you think could be improved. Of course, it's also good to mention what you thought they did well.

**KEEP ALL YOUR FINISHING MEDALS WHERE YOU CAN SEE THEM:** If you have a separate closet or closet area with all your running clothes, that's a perfect spot for your medals. Or hang them on a big hook next to your bedroom dresser. Preferably they should be in plain view so that they'll motivate you and bring back great memories every time you glance at them.

**SAVE YOUR RACE NUMBERS, TOO:** Actually, you can get pretty creative with these. I've known runners who have essentially used their race numbers as wallpaper and covered entire closet walls with them. Others have sewn them together to create jackets or quilts. You might also write on your race numbers the date of the race, the time you ran and your place, and a short personal note on how the race went for you.

**TAKE AN EASY DAY OF RECOVERY FOR EVERY MILE YOU RACE:** This is a great rule I first heard years ago. For example, if you run a half marathon, which is 13.1 miles, take around 13 easy days after the race to recover. For a marathon, you get 26 days—almost a month! Easy doesn't mean no running at all, though that's probably fine the first few days after the event. Rather, just keep away from hard runs (intervals, *fartlek*, etc.), superhilly runs, or long runs during your recovery time. Only easy running allowed.

**BUY AND FRAME A RACE PICTURE OF YOURSELF:** They're not that expensive, and they make great mementos. Perfect for the wall at work, or on your desk, as a nice reminder of your exploits.

**BE PROUD OF YOUR RACING ACHIEVEMENTS, BUT DON'T EXPECT YOUR COWORKERS TO "GET IT":** Sometimes runners can get a little carried away talking about their running and racing. That's fine among friends, but at work it's probably best to stay low-key. No one wants to be a bore!

**BE SMART ABOUT THE RACES YOU SELECT:** Okay, you did progressively better in a series of 5K races in the summer, so now your training partner says, "Hey, let's run a full marathon!" For 10 bonus points, what is your answer? Good for you. Sure, go ahead and applaud his or her enthusiasm and the long-term goal of running the Big Kahuna, but it's smart to work up to the marathon by first tackling a half marathon. That's a plenty big challenge itself.

# GET YOUR HEAD READY TO RACE

*As director of high performance at Nike and sports psychologist for the Nike Oregon Project, Darren Treasure, PhD, has been working with me on the mental aspects of running for several years. Here's a detailed psych-up plan guaranteed to get you stoked and focused for your next race, courtesy of Darren Treasure.*

Kara is totally professional in her approach to training, competition, rest/sleep, nutrition, family, and social life. She takes responsibility for the choices she makes and recognizes that almost everything she does each day will ultimately affect her race performance.

For all runners, planning is the key to performing your best. The planning process can last anywhere from a few weeks to a few years. In Kara's case, we are in the middle of a four-year planning process that began immediately after she finished ninth in the 5,000m at the Beijing Olympics. If all goes well, it will end at the conclusion of the London Olympic Marathon in 2012.

209

# The Weeks Leading Up to the Race

These weeks are particularly important for laying the mental ground-work for your race. Consider the following strategies:

- **Practice positive self-talk.** It's important to understand that what we say triggers images in our mind that affect our emotions and behavior. Learning to control your self-talk before a race will help you develop a positive mindset about your running in general and the race you are preparing for.
- **Develop a list of affirmation statements.** These statements are designed to be both aspirational (what you hope for) and inspirational. To start, choose four statements (e.g., "I am strong," "I am a fierce competitor") and repeat them three to four times a day. This may feel a little awkward or silly at first, but stick with them. They will help you develop a positive mindset. Another good idea is to post your affirmations in places where you'll see them so that they'll be a constant reminder of who you want to be as a runner.
- **Visualize for 5 minutes a day.** Do this in a quiet place when you are calm and your mind is ready to receive the images you are creating. Remember that what you see/feel is what you will get. If you can see and feel yourself being the runner you want to be, there is a far greater probability that you will be this person.
- **Take care of the nuts and bolts.** Especially if you need to travel to your race, make sure you're all set regarding travel, accommodations, and restaurants. You don't want any last-minute stressors affecting your race.

# The Day/Night Before the Race

This critical period may require two different routines—one for home races and one for away races. That said, the more similar you can make the two routines the better.

- **Check out the venue.** Visit and potentially walk/jog important sections of the course. Spend some time at the end of the course; close your eyes and imagine what it will feel like to finish tomorrow's race and achieve the goal(s) you have set for yourself.

- **Go out for a meal—but keep things lighthearted.** Remember—no trying any exotic new cuisine! Stick with foods that have worked in the past, that you know your stomach can handle. Before major competitions, Kara eats Italian with her husband, coach, and me. There is no talk of the race. It is simply a relaxed affair that makes her feel comfortable and confident.
- **"See" it once more.** Back home or back at the hotel, do a visualization session that includes a focus on race strategy.
- **Get things set.** Have your race clothes and equipment in order and set out for the next morning. Repeat affirmation statements.
- **Relax, then hit the sack.** Indulge in relaxation activity—watching TV, reading, viewing a movie—anything that will help you sleep and to simply chill. Oh, and even if you have your own alarm clock, ask for a wake-up call!

## The Morning of the Race

Depending on the race start, be prepared to make adjustments to your normal routine. When Kara ran the New York City Marathon in 2008, she had to be on the bus at 5:30 A.M. for a 9:10 A.M. start. She actually took a pillow and blanket on the bus with her so that she could sleep a little more on the way to and before the start. In contrast, the 10,000-meter race at the 2008 Olympic Trials in Eugene took place at 9:30 P.M. Regardless, as you get closer to your start time, your routine needs to be consistent and well rehearsed. However, it should not be so inflexible that a change or logistical slip-up completely undermines the routine. Here's a simple four-step routine for those critical minutes before the start:

1. 30 minutes before the race start: Do a supereasy 10-minute jog.
2. 20 minutes before the start: Do 5 minutes of stretching, then 5 minutes of strides.

3. 10 minutes before the start: Do a little more jogging, plus positive visualization.

4. 5 minutes before the start: Move to the start area.

Routines work for three main reasons:

1. They help you block out distractions and create a positive mindset.

2. They provide a sense of familiarity that is calming.

3. They provide a framework that ensures consistent preparation, which in turn leads to better performance.

# During the Race

- **Be ready to answer the tough questions.** Kara has adopted a simple mental approach to her races. Namely, she expects the best but is always prepared for the worst. She knows there will be moments during the race when her conditioning, her toughness, and her confidence will be tested.

- **Remember the power of the word.** One of the strategies we have worked on is the development of a power word. For this to be most effective, it's best to practice with this word in training as well, before your race. For the 2007 season, Kara chose the word *fighter,* which was perfect for where she was in her psychological development. It reflected her desire to want to fight for acceptance as a world-class athlete. She used this word in moments in races that year when she needed to dig deep and fight through a period of adversity. Kara's power word has changed over time, but she always has one.

- **Keep the focus on you and not the runners around you.** Even at the elite level, this is important. I always say to Kara that she becomes world class when she focuses on herself. She becomes less than that when she focuses on or worries about others.

# The World's Simplest Race-Training Plans

With each of the three plans outlined here, you only have to run three days a week. Your first workout each week will be an easy run, your second workout will be a hard run (with effort), and your third workout—normally run on the weekend when you have more time—will be a long run. Three workouts—easy, hard, long.

For more advanced runners who want to do more or who are aiming for a time goal in each of these race distances, all you need to do is add more running on the other four days of the week. Just be sure that you run easy, though one additional hard run would be fine, to give you two total for the week. Otherwise, easy does it. It's the additional mileage that will boost your fitness, and easy runs do that just as well as hard or long runs. Better in fact, as there's less risk of injury or over-training.

- **Point #1:** As you'll see, each of the schedules lists workouts in miles. If you know your average minutes-per-mile training pace, feel free to convert your training schedule to minutes of running rather than miles of running. Many runners prefer to run by minutes, and that's fine. Either way works.
- **Point #2:** As for how much running you should be doing at the point you start each of the schedules, that's simple. You'll need to be at the point where you're doing at least the equivalent of what's required in week 1. Be careful to arrive at that point gradually; you don't want to make the leap from nothing (absolute beginner) to the listed plan, even the 5K plan, which has the easiest starting point.
- **Point #3:** The training schedules each have you doing your running on Tuesdays, Thursdays, and Sundays. You don't have to stick to these days. If running three days a week is better for you on Mondays, Wednesdays, and Saturdays, that's totally okay. Really, as long as you have at least one and preferably two days between your hard and long runs, you'll be fine with whichever days you

choose. Just try to keep it consistent from week to week so that you can get into a routine.

Before getting to the schedules themselves, here are some quick notes on each of the three runs:

- **Tuesday easy runs:** Just like it says—easy effort. Conversational pace. You should finish these with no huffing and puffing, no problem. The point is pure cardio: extend your endurance, burn calories, strengthen your legs, boost your confidence. These runs are easy but very important. So don't discount them as mere "junk miles," to use an old running term.

- **Thursday hard runs:** Endurance is the key requirement for distance races, and you can build endurance simply by increasing the length of your once-a-week long run. Adding a shorter hard run each week just gets you there faster. It's also excellent for burning calories, improving running form, increasing your ability to process oxygen, and boosting mental toughness.

  No need to do these all-out, and by the way, the entire run will not be hard! On each of your hard run days, you'll warm up with easy running first, then you'll do a series of hard segments (with easy running in between each segment), then cool down with more easy running. How hard are the hard segments? Run them at "tempo" pace. In the simplest terms, this is midway between your easy jogging pace and your sprinting pace. At the end of your last hard segment, you should feel like you could do at least one more if you had to—if not two or three more. You will know you did the workout just right when you feel energized and pumped up about what you just did, not exhausted.

- **Sunday long runs:** As with your easy runs, these are very straightforward, just like the label implies. You'll want to run them at your easy run pace—if not easier!—as it's simply about covering the territory. These do everything your easy runs do for you, but with more emphasis on endurance. As such, they are far and away the most important training component for the half marathon. As mentioned, these can take some time out of your day—up to one to two hours as you get close to your half-marathon race—so it usually works best to schedule them for the weekend. It also helps to do them with a training partner who can accompany you for at least part of the way.

## The World's Simplest 5K Training Plan (6 Weeks)

|  | Tuesday | Thursday | Sunday |
|---|---|---|---|
| Week 1 | 1 mile | 2 X ¼ miles* | 2 miles |
| Week 2 | 1 | 2 X ¼ | 2 |
| Week 3 | 2 | 3 X ¼ | 2 |
| Week 4 | 2 | 3 X ¼ | 2 |
| Week 5 | 2 | 4 X ¼ | 2 |
| Week 6 | 2 | 2 X ¼ | 5K race |

## The World's Simplest 10K Training Plan (9 Weeks)

|  | Tuesday | Thursday | Sunday |
|---|---|---|---|
| Week 1 | 2 miles | 3 X ¼ miles† | 3 miles |
| Week 2 | 2 | 3 X ¼ | 3 |
| Week 3 | 2 | 4 X ¼ | 4 |
| Week 4 | 2 | 4 X ¼ | 4 |
| Week 5 | 3 | 4 X ¼ | 4 |

* On each of your hard days, always start with 1 mile of very easy running, followed by the specified number of hard segments. Between your hard segments, do ¼ mile of brisk walking. Always finish with ½ mile of easy cooldown. Thus, on your first hard day, you'll do: 1 mile easy, ¼ mile hard, ¼ mile walk, ¼ mile hard, ½ mile cooldown.

† On each of your hard days, always start with 1 mile of very easy running, followed by the specified number of hard segments, always with ¼ mile of very easy running between the hard segments. Always finish with ½ mile easy cooldown. Thus, on your first hard day, you'll do: 1 mile easy, ¼ mile hard, ¼ mile easy, ¼ mile hard, ¼ mile easy, ¼ mile hard, ½ mile cooldown.

|         | Tuesday | Thursday | Sunday   |
|---------|---------|----------|----------|
| Week 6  | 3       | 4 X ¼    | 5        |
| Week 7  | 3       | 5 X ¼    | 5        |
| Week 8  | 2       | 5 X ¼    | 5        |
| Week 9  | 2       | 2 X ¼    | 10K race |

## The World's Simplest Half-Marathon Training Plan (12 Weeks)

|          | Tuesday | Thursday     | Sunday             |
|----------|---------|--------------|--------------------|
| Week 1   | 3 miles | 2 X ½ miles* | 4 miles            |
| Week 2   | 3       | 2 X ½        | 5                  |
| Week 3   | 3       | 2 X ½        | 6                  |
| Week 4   | 3       | 2 X ½        | 7                  |
| Week 5   | 4       | 3 X ½        | 5                  |
| Week 6   | 4       | 3 X ½        | 8                  |
| Week 7   | 4       | 3 X ½        | 6                  |
| Week 8   | 4       | 3 X ½        | 9                  |
| Week 9   | 5       | 4 X ½        | 7                  |
| Week 10  | 5       | 4 X ½        | 10                 |
| Week 11  | 5       | 4 X ½        | 5                  |
| Week 12  | 5       | 2 X ½        | Half-marathon race |

* On each of your hard days, always start with 1 mile of very easy running, followed by the specified number of hard segments, always with ½ mile of very easy running between the hard segments. Always finish with 1 mile easy cooldown. Thus, on your first hard day, you'll do: 1 mile easy, ½ mile hard, ½ mile easy, ½ mile hard, 1 mile cooldown.

# Fun Races to Try

Your standard neighborhood 5K or 10K road race is a blast. These races are all over the place, easy to find and enter, and they're great for keeping you motivated and for testing your fitness. But you have a lot of other inspiring race options to choose from as well.

- **Women-only races:** The biggest of these is the Susan G. Komen Race for the Cure 5K series, which raises money and awareness for breast cancer. But there are all sorts of local women-only races as well, including the Baltimore Women's Classic 5K, the Freihofer's Run for Women 5K, the Idaho Women's Fitness Celebration 5K, the *More* magazine Half Marathon, the New York Mini 10K, and the Nike Women's Marathon and Half Marathon.

- **Hill/mountain races:** You don't run these for time (slow!), but rather to say you survived them. What a feeling afterward—it'll stay with you a lifetime. Three longtime classics are the Falmouth Road Race on Cape Cod (challenging), the Pikes Peak Ascent (brutal), and the Mount Washington Road Race (off the charts).

- **Trail races:** A wonderful get-away-from-it-all adventure, a trail race is way different from a road race. Quieter, more solitary, more introspective. Sometimes it's just you and nature for extended periods of the race—amazing. For a listing of trail races nationwide, check out the American Trail Running Association's website at trailrunner.com.

- **Mile races:** Who says you need to be out there racing for 30 minutes, an hour, or longer? You have plenty of short-and-sweet mile races—normally called "road miles"—out there to choose from. Many are fun runs attached to longer races, but some are the featured event. That's 6 to 12 minutes of hard racing (depending on your speed) and you're done for the day!

- **Stair-climbing races:** The Empire State Building Run-Up is probably the oldest of these fun but crazy events (thirty-fourth annual in 2011), but you can also do a stair-climb race up the Willis Tower (formerly Sears Tower) in Chicago, the U.S. Bank Tower in Los Angeles, and many other challenging venues besides. Just beware of the thigh burn. The Empire State version takes in 86 floors and 1,576 steps.

# CHAPTER 8

# RUNNING A MARATHON

I never seriously considered running a marathon until after I ran my first half marathon, the Great North Run in England, on a whim in 2007. If I told you that I had the time of my life racing 13.1 miles and that I finished the race hungry to go even farther, I would be lying. On the contrary, it hurt more than any other race I had run. But I ran so well—defeating the marathon world record holder and running the fastest half marathon ever by an American—that I came away from it thinking that I might have a future in the marathon. I was suddenly intrigued by distance running's ultimate challenge.

Still, I was in no hurry to run my first 26.2-miler. I figured I would wait until after Adam and I had our first child. But fate intervened. Shortly after I returned home from England, I received an invitation from Mary Wittenberg, president of the New York Road Runners, to watch that year's race as a special guest. Mary always works hard to lure up-and-coming runners to her race, and I guess she had marked me as the next up-and-comer.

Fatigue from a whirlwind year almost persuaded me to turn down the invitation, but curiosity got the better of me and I accepted it at the last minute. It's funny how often we make life-changing decisions with ambivalence at the last minute.

Paula Radcliffe had run the Great North Run as a tune-up race for the New York City Marathon. I did not come away from our head-to-head match-up with any illusions that my beating her made me the better runner, but if I had, watching her run in New York would have cured me of them. Her performance was awe-inspiring—and a little intimidating.

I had a seat on a truck that traveled just in front of the lead women from the start line to the finish line. Also on the truck was Kim Smith, a rising runner from New Zealand who Mary Wittenberg was also trying to lure to the next year's New York City Marathon. It takes a while for even Paula Radcliffe to run a marathon, so I assumed that Kim and I would spend a lot of time chatting and getting to know each other. Instead, we barely spoke after the first mile. We were both completely riveted by Paula's performance.

What amazed me most was how hard Paula worked the whole way. Although I knew athletes like Paula ran marathons very fast, I still viewed the marathon as a more leisurely affair than the track races I was used to running. But there was nothing leisurely about how Paula Radcliffe ran the 2007 New York City Marathon. She and Gete Wami of Ethiopia started so fast that they had separated themselves from the other elite women after only 4 miles. Paula led, with Gete shadowing her for the next 21.5 miles. With less than a mile to go, Paula's relentless near-course-record pace finally became too much for Gete, who decided that second place wasn't so bad as Paula pulled away for the win.

It was one of the most stunning displays of pure toughness I had ever seen. I admired it. I envied it. I wanted it. Just like that I was desperately eager to run a marathon, not because I thought it was a great career move, but because I wanted to see myself the way I knew Paula must see herself. I wanted to be that tough.

I shared my feelings with Alberto and he expressed his support. Without wasting another day, I began negotiations to run the New York City Marathon the following November. What made these plans a bit tricky was that I hoped to qualify for and run in the Olympics in the summer, and the second and last of my two events, the 10,000m, would take place a mere ten weeks before the marathon. And the first of those ten weeks would have to be used for recovery and the last for tapering. But Alberto assured me that the eight weeks in the middle would be plenty of time to add enough endurance to my track speed to set me up for a successful first marathon, provided I managed my expectations and raced to compete and learn rather than to win and break records.

The Olympics happen only once every four years. Elite runners can race two or three good marathons every year. So Alberto and I decided to stay focused exclusively on the Olympics until they were over and to modify my training very little in anticipation of New York. Once Beijing was behind me, everything changed. After a one-week break, my very first marathon training run was an 18-miler, the longest run of my life. Alberto rode a bike alongside me. Thirteen miles into it, he suddenly pulled over.

"Stop! Stop! Stop!" he said. I stopped. He unzipped his backpack, pulled out a weight vest, and handed it to me. "Put this on."

So this is how it's going to be, I thought.

And that's how it was. Those eight weeks were a continuous grind. I often felt as if I was wearing that weight vest even when I wasn't. Alberto made sure I got enough recovery to keep my body from falling apart completely, but I was tired constantly. I loved it, though. I really enjoyed the all-consuming nature of the experience. Plus, I was the only one on my team training for a marathon. It was my own special thing.

The nearer race day came, the more nervous I got. I barely survived my longest training run, a 23-miler. How the heck was I going to make it 26.2 miles? My anxiety became a near panic when we arrived

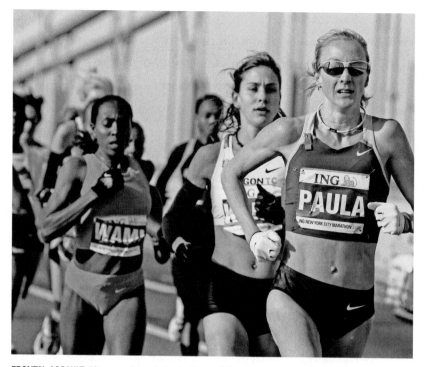

**FRONTAL ASSAULT:** After a much-needed calm-down talk from marathon world record holder Paula Radcliffe on the bus ride to the start of the 2008 ING New York City Marathon, I tuck in behind her on the Verrazano-Narrows Bridge during the early miles.

in New York and I saw how much hype surrounded my participation in the race. It's one thing not to make it to the finish line. It's another thing to fall short with seemingly the whole world watching.

Alberto talked me off the ledge. "Everything has gone perfectly," he said. "Do you realize that never happens? You haven't had a single setback. You're ready."

Early on race morning, all of the elite runners were herded onto a bus that carried us to the start area on the Verrazano-Narrows Bridge. Neither Adam nor Alberto could go with me. I felt alone and scared. My only comfort was a big, puffy comforter Alberto had bought me the night before to keep me warm in the November morning chill. (He tries to think of everything!) I buried myself underneath it and tried to hide my tears.

Paula Radcliffe, who had returned to New York to defend her title, sat down beside me. Seeing my distress, she started a completely one-sided conversation that filled the whole hour of the drive. I was humbled by her generosity. Here she was under twice the pressure I had to deal with, yet she still was willing and able to get outside of herself and talk her throat dry to calm me down.

The bus dumped us onto the cold, wind-exposed bridge, where we had nothing to do but shiver and wait. My fear was literally nauseating. I sent Adam some self-pitying texts. Then, all of a sudden, we were called to the start line. Where had the time gone? I had only completed half my warm-up. *This is a disaster!*

Nothing cures prerace terrors like the start of the race. Once I was running, I felt fine. It helped that a slow 6:30 first mile allowed me to gently ease my body and mind into my first marathon. I fell into a comfortable rhythm with the lead pack, closely marking Paula. The first half of the race went by surprisingly quickly, yet it was long enough for my thoughts to wander a bit. I thought a lot about my dad. Only when I talked to my mom after the race did I discover that his presence in my mind was most powerful as the race took us through Queens, where our family had lived for two years.

I knew the race would not remain comfortable forever. My calves began to hurt as we ran over the lonely Queensboro Bridge into Manhattan between the 15- and 16-mile marks. Doubt followed the pain into my mind. Alberto and some other New York City Marathon veterans had told me to expect to get a motivational boost from the massive crowds of spectators lining the long, straight corridor of First Avenue, and I did. Trouble was, Paula got an even bigger boost and threw down a couple of sub-5:20 miles.

I can't do this, I thought, and let her drift away. I wasn't being defeatist. I knew I really couldn't keep up with her and would be a fool to try. By now the pain in my legs had crept into my knees and above. There were other problems. I kept fumbling with the bottles of fluid set out for me at aid stations, dropping them, and thus getting nothing to drink. As I became dehydrated, I began to cramp. And what little I did drink wouldn't stay down. I threw up bright orange geysers of sport drink a couple of times.

Despite all of these issues, I kept my competitive mindset and remembered the example of toughness Paula had set for me a year before. Paula and Ludmila Petrova were ahead of me. Gete Wami and Dire Tune were with me. Five runners, three podium spots. *I have to get that third spot. I have to get away now!*

I surged hard. Or at least I thought I did at the time. When I later studied my mile splits, I discovered that my pace was perfectly even during this part of the race. That's the marathon for you: You think you're speeding up, but you're just hanging on. You think you're hanging on, but you're slowing down. You think you're slowing down, but you're *really* slowing down. In any case, whatever I did was enough to drop the other girls, and I found myself alone in third place.

No matter how well you prepare for it, the difficulty of the last few miles of your first marathon can be shocking. I was in such agony as I grinded my way toward the finish line in Central Park that I actively searched for a discreet spot where I could drop out with only a half mile left to go in the race. The thought of continuing to run even three minutes longer was unbearable. The only reason I didn't drop out—or so it seemed at the time—was that there were too many darn witnesses.

Adam gave me a big hug and a hearty congratulations after I crossed the finish line. My third-place finish was the best by an American woman in the New York City Marathon since 1983, and my time of 2:25:53 was the fastest debut marathon ever by an American woman.

"Everything went wrong," I told Adam sulkily. This was far from true, but it was how I felt at the moment. I knew I could have done much better if not for the missed bottles, the cramping, and the vomit-

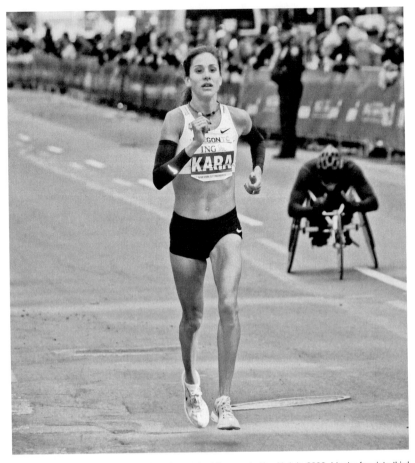

**LONE RANGER:** After jousting with others for much of the race in New York in 2008, I broke free into third place as the finish line nears.

ing, not to mention the energy-wasting way I had insisted on following Paula's every move as long as I could. Despite the misery I had just experienced, I couldn't wait for my next chance to run a marathon. Although I had run like a rookie, I felt amazingly at home in the race, as though I had finally discovered what I'd really been born for. Discovering the marathon was like falling in love with running all over again. I had found my best and favorite place in the sport.

# SUREFIRE STRATEGIES TO HELP YOU RUN THE BEST 26.2-MILER OF YOUR LIFE

came to the marathon relatively late in my running career. It was the 2008 ING New York City Marathon, and I was thirty. At that point, I'd been a runner for eighteen years.

Which is why I'm allowed to say . . . take your time before committing to this marathon thing. They're not going anywhere, so no rush to do one. I think it's smart to take a few years to build up your running endurance before trying 26.2 miles. Sometimes I think there's too much emphasis these days on doing the marathon as your first race, courtesy of so many "we'll get you there!" programs. Most of the time things turn out just fine—I'm not trying to be a killjoy here—but to me it seems like a lot to ask of yourself.

Meanwhile, you can get your toes wet in shorter races. The half marathon has been gaining in popularity for years now, and I think it's a great distance. It's a big challenge, but it doesn't require the time, commitment, and training of a marathon. The 10K and 5K distances are fun, too.

Then again, maybe you *are* ready for the big enchilada. Maybe this is the year to do one. If you get excited just thinking about the prospect, well, that tells you something.

If a marathon is in your near future, check out the marathon tips on the following pages. They're appropriate for first-timers and veterans alike. You may want to look at Chapter 7 as well. Many of those tips apply to the marathon.

**TRAIN FOR A MARATHON THE SIMPLE WAY:** You'll find a really basic marathon-training plan later in this chapter, but you can get even more basic than that: two short runs during the week (5 miles each or so) and a long run on the weekend. Extend the long run by 1 mile a week until you reach 10 miles, then by 2 miles a week until you reach 20 miles. At which point you'll be ready to run your marathon. Be sure you run short and easy for two or three weeks before the race.

**KNOW YOUR END GOAL (RUNNING A MARATHON!), BUT TRAIN DAY TO DAY:** For first-timers especially, but really for anyone training for a marathon, glancing ahead at your training schedule can be seriously daunting. It's the long runs that are the most scary. Okay, 10 miles isn't so bad for a training run, but 15? 18? 20? New marathoners have a tough time imagining themselves going that far when it's not even the race yet, which is why it is so important to not look ahead at the schedule very often. Just deal with the week you're in, and be determined to complete each of the runs scheduled for that week. When that week is done, look at the next week. And so on. You'll get there. Steady as she goes.

**PICK THE RIGHT MARATHON FOR YOU:** There are hundreds of great marathons in the United States and hundreds more around the world. Some get fifty thousand participants. Some get fifty. Some are hilly. Some are flat. Some are hot. Some are cold. Point being, it's important to pick one that suits you, which can make all the difference in terms of what you get out of it. To help you decide, here are the pros and cons of three main types.

### Big-City Marathons
- **Pros:** an event as much as a race; lots of fun; lots of excitement; more spectators; plenty of people to run with the entire way; good in-race entertainment (e.g., bands); good vacation possibility for you and your family

227

- **Cons:** more expense (the race and the city); can be a hassle picking up your race number; can be a hassle getting to the start and back from the finish; crowded conditions for at least the first several miles

### Small-City Marathons

- **Pros:** less expense (the race and the city); easier to get to the start and back from the finish; no race crowds to keep you from a PR; easier to find lodgings; easier to focus on the race itself
- **Cons:** less all-around excitement; fewer spectators; occasionally "spotty" course management; fewer runners to run with; occasionally less than stellar in-race entertainment

### Rural/Scenic Marathons

- **Pros:** rural and scenic (!); less crowd hassle; accommodating "mom-and-pop" race organization
- **Cons:** can be tough to reach; less excitement; fewer runners to run with; occasionally spotty course management; usually less impressive race goody bag; fewer lodging options

**TRAIN FOR YOUR SPECIFIC MARATHON:** Certain aspects of marathon training apply to all marathons. You need to do your long runs, for instance. And you need to eat right, get plenty of sleep, and taper for two to three weeks beforehand. But there are some key ways you can and should tailor your training to suit the marathon you choose. So check the race site and see what the course is like (hilly or flat, paved or trail, etc.), what typical race-day temperatures are likely to be, the elevation of the course, and so on. Several of these factors will change how you train for it.

**MAKE SURE YOU DON'T SKIMP ON THE LONG STUFF:** For the great majority of runners, the weekly or biweekly long run is far and away the most important part of marathon training. And again, for most people it

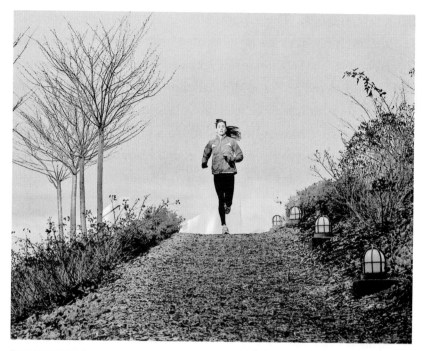

**THE LONG VERSION:** Since stepping up to the marathon distance in 2008, I have made long runs a steady part of my training diet. As they'll need to be for you, if you decide to tackle 26.2.

doesn't really matter how fast or slow you do it; it's simply about doing it. It's about being on your feet and moving forward for two or three hours. Its important for you physically to do this, but also mentally, so come race day, you'll be completely confident of success.

**DO IT FOR THE RIGHT REASONS:** Training for a marathon takes a lot of time, energy, and commitment. You don't want to make that kind of commitment unless the goal of running a marathon really makes sense for you. New runners sometimes sign up for their first marathon before they're ready just because they have friends who run marathons. Experienced runners often run marathons because they think they won't be considered serious athletes if they run only the shorter races they prefer. These are not good reasons to run marathons. The reason you're running one needs to come from the heart.

**RUNNING A MARATHON**

**SET A REALISTIC GOAL:** The marathon loves to crush the ambitions of first-timers. It doesn't care how talented or fit you are or how much success you've had in shorter races. Haile Gebrselassie is the current men's world record holder in the marathon (2:03:59!), but he got his butt kicked in his first three marathons before he mastered it. So it's important to set a conservative goal for your first marathon. Focus on finishing, having a positive experience, and learning things that will enable you to run your best marathon in the future.

# I LOVE THIS QUOTE

Now I want to find out, How fast can I go? Can I run under 2:20 for a marathon? Okay, if I don't do it, it's not a catastrophe, but the question still hasn't been answered. I want to take a fair shot at finding an answer.

—Uta Pippig, 1994 Boston and
ING New York City Marathon Winner

I love this quote because it is exactly how I feel. One of my goals is to run 2:18. If I never run 2:18, my life will go on, but I want to know in all of my heart that I did everything I could. I want to know if I am capable of this goal.

**BUT THINK THROUGH A PLAN B AS WELL:** Too many marathoners have trained like dogs for several months, only for marathon day to come and it's *way* hotter than it was supposed to be. What do these marathoners do then? All too frequently, they stick with the original plan and hope for the best. Not a good strategy. The crazy-heat-on-race-day scenario requires some advance planning, such as having an alternate marathon to run perhaps a month after the hot one. With that marathon to look forward to, you can relax, slow down, and use the hot marathon as a long training run—complete with fluid replacement throughout. (If you don't end up needing that backup race, let the event organizers know, and consider your entry fee a donation to the race.)

**ALLOW ENOUGH TIME TO TRAIN, BUT NOT TOO MUCH:** What does it mean to be in training for a marathon? It means you are gradually and steadily increasing your training load to build the fitness you need to run (or race) 26.2 miles. Runners at all levels can only increase their training load so long before they get injured, overtired, or psychologically burned out. So, while you want to allow plenty of time to increase your running gradually to prepare for a marathon, there's such a thing as training too long. If you feel you need more than twelve to sixteen weeks to prepare for a marathon, then you're probably not ready for a marathon. Devote ten to twelve weeks to training for a half marathon instead, then take a break and build up for a marathon.

**FOCUS ON BUILDING CONFIDENCE:** Runners typically think about training in purely physical terms, but I like to think about it as a process of confidence building. When you train for a marathon, think about what you will need to do to be confident of a successful race, then do it. How long should your longest run be? How much running should you do at your goal pace? How much recovery should you build into your plan so that you feel strong for your important workouts? Let your sense of confidence guide you in making these decisions. Once you've made them—and followed through on them—confidence will follow.

**BE PREPARED FOR SETBACKS:** Something—usually more than one thing—always goes wrong when you train for a marathon. At the very least, you will probably find that at some point you have trouble recovering from your workouts and have to take a few unplanned recovery days to restore your energy. In addition, you can expect aches and pains and perhaps one or more small injuries requiring additional unscheduled rest. If you suffer no greater setbacks than these in your marathon training, call it a success. The secret to dealing with such setbacks is to expect them and respond to them quickly and decisively without panicking.

## DEAR KARA

**I've done three marathons. In each one, I feel great until 17 or 18 miles, then it's a death march. Just awful. I do plenty of long runs in training—several of 20 miles, in fact—but do you think I need to do them faster? I go pretty slow.**

Ahh, the infamous wall that all marathoners hit around that 17- to 20-mile mark. I have hit that, too. I do think that it might be prudent to do every third long run or so at a faster pace. Not necessarily race pace, but make sure that you are working hard. You don't have to do every long run like that, but it will help your stamina when you run harder and longer on race day. Also, take a look at your nutrition. Are you getting enough electrolytes during the race? If you aren't replacing enough during the marathon, you are sure to be totally depleted by the 17- to 20-mile mark. Make sure you are getting enough calories during the race.

**PRACTICE YOUR NUTRITION:** Race nutrition is vital to success in the marathon. Find out which sport drink is being served at aid stations in your next marathon and practice with it in training to get comfortable with it. But if you have a sensitive stomach (like me), you might want to play it safe and drink water, using carbohydrate gels that you carry with you to provide the carbs and sodium your body needs. In that case, it's this routine you'll want to practice in training, especially on your long runs.

**KEEP UP WITH THE SPEEDY STUFF:** This will keep your form sharp. Even at the world-class level, marathon runners often neglect their speed, and as a result they develop "pace lock." That is, they get stuck in third gear, having lost their fourth and fifth gears—then their form starts to deteriorate. Probably the best and easiest way to do speedwork is to continue doing shorter races. I look at it this way: The faster I can run a 5K, the faster I can run a 10K. The faster I can run a 10K, the faster I can run a half marathon. And the faster I can run a half marathon, the faster I can run a marathon. Makes sense, right?

**GROOVE YOUR GOAL PACE:** Perhaps the most important ingredient for success in the marathon is a high level of comfort with and efficiency at your goal pace. Your body and mind need to know that pace intimately. That means your marathon training has to include a lot of running at your goal pace.

**TAKE THE LONG VIEW:** It takes several years to develop the fitness you need to run your best marathon. Try to be patient and enjoy the process. I don't expect to run my best marathon for another three years. And while on one level I can't wait to get there, I'm more focused on the stepping-stones. It's not exactly instant gratification, but who runs marathons for instant gratification? That's what ice cream is for!

# DEAR KARA

**I've been a runner for twenty years. I'm forty-two now and I've never run a marathon. I want to do it, but I'm scared I won't have the endurance and will crash and burn. Any advice?**

It is a big thing to ask of yourself, but you can do it. Remember, you can always slow down and walk. The point is to keep moving forward. Take your time in training for one, but don't put pressure on yourself to run any certain time. Oprah ran a marathon; you can, too!

**BE SAFE AND SMART DURING YOUR TAPER PERIOD:** Your marathon taper is the last two to three weeks before the race when you back way off on your mileage and intensity, which allows your body and mind to rest up for the task ahead. Some runners have a tough time with this critical period, as they start thinking they're losing their hard-won fitness. Just relax! Keep running, but just do a lot less of it. Fight the urge to run long or hard. Two to three weeks isn't enough time to improve your fitness in any significant way, but it *is* enough time to get yourself injured.

**TAKE TIME FOR THE RACE EXPO:** Make no mistake, running a marathon is a big deal, so make the most of the experience. Marathon race expos happen the day before the race (big races have multiday expos), and you can browse the booths for information and occasional free samples (!) on all sorts of running products, from energy bars and sport drinks to treadmills and body-fat calculators. The expo is where you pick up your race number as well. Bring your family and friends with you, and be sure to buy at least one memento with the marathon race logo on it.

**RUN WITH A PACE GROUP:** A lot of half marathons have these now, but pace groups are even more key in a marathon, where even pacing—not to mention in-race camaraderie—is so important. An experienced pace-group leader takes you through the entire race at an even pace. All you and your fellow group members need to do is stay with him or her. These groups don't cost anything, and you don't usually have to sign up. When you get to the start, look for the pace group that's planning to run the time you're planning to run, then run with them. Presto—a solo sport becomes a team sport, and you benefit from the group energy.

**DON'T OVERDRESS:** Most marathons start in the early morning to take maximum advantage of cool temperatures. That's fine, but don't make the mistake of thinking it'll be chilly the entire race and wearing tights and a long-sleeve T-shirt. A good rule of thumb is that you should feel slightly cool for the first mile of the race. If that's the case, you've dressed properly. Remember, you can always put clothes back on (wrapping them around your waist is fine), but you can only take so many off. For all but the chilliest marathons, shorts and a top is the way to go.

**PROTECT YOUR EYES AND SKIN:** Another tip from the racing chapter, but it's so important in a marathon, as you're out there for three, four, five, sometimes six hours or more. That's a long time to be in the sun without protection. In fact, you may want to bring sunscreen along with you so that you can reapply it halfway through the race. A hat with a brim and sunglasses are a must.

## ON THE CONTRARY

This may seem crazy, but I don't wear a watch during my road races. I think that obsessing over the time can take away from your performance. I see the clocks at each mile or kilometer marker and I take little mental notes. But I really just try to focus on what I'm doing and how I'm feeling. I use the clocks as a very loose guide and really try to just listen to my body.

**SAVOR RACE DAY:** Well-known running columnist and "penguin runner" John Bingham has a funny way to describe how he feels when the marathon starting gun goes off. He says he wants to take his time and take it all in! "I didn't train all that time just to come here and get it over with as fast as I can," he says. There's something to that. Good things shouldn't be rushed. Running your best is important, absolutely, and I think every runner should try pushing as hard as she can in a marathon at least once in her life. It is incredibly satisfying and memorable. But taking the time to savor every minute is powerful as well.

235

**DOUBLE-KNOT YOUR SHOES:** It really stinks to have your shoes come untied in a marathon. If it happens near the beginning, you risk getting trampled. If it happens farther in, it can be tough to bend down to re-tie! When you're lined up at the start, do a quick check of everything. Socks not bunching up? Ponytail tight? Sports bra in position? Fannypack adjusted? Stopwatch reset to zero?

**GO REAL EASY FOR THE FIRST FEW MILES:** Hey, 26.2 miles is a long way—you'll get there eventually. Seriously, chances are you're going to feel really good those first few miles of the marathon (or any race distance, for that matter) with all that training behind you and the crowds and bands lifting your spirits. So make a conscious effort to hold back. Conserve energy. Rein it way in until at least the 10-mile mark, if not the 20-mile mark! Alberto told me that when he ran his first marathon, he got about 10 miles into the race and then asked the guy next to him, "When does it get hard?" The other runner answered, "Just wait."

**BE MINDFUL OF THOSE AROUND YOU:** There can be a lot of jostling in the first couple miles. People sprinting past who lined up too far back. Race walkers coming back to you who started too far forward. Basically, it's just a lot of people sharing a sometimes-narrow road. Leave ample space ahead of you so that you don't trip those in front. Keep your hands ready and alert to catch yourself should you get tripped or jostled. And always do a quick head-check before shifting left or right.

**DON'T START OUT TOO FAST!** This is probably mistake number one for newbie marathoners, in part because the beginning of the race really should feel very easy. When it does feel easy, runners figure, "Wow, today is my day. I'm feeling great. I'm going to go faster!" Which they do—until they hit mile 15, at which point they start kicking themselves for going too fast early on. So don't make that mistake. Whatever pace you have trained to maintain in the race, stick to it no matter what. If you feel great at mile 20, fine, pick up the pace. But not until then.

**RUN "NEGATIVE SPLITS":** This means running the second half of the race faster than the first. It's a great habit to get into, and you invariably feel much better (mentally *and* physically) during and after the race if you can pull it off. Of course, to make it work, you need to follow the advice in the previous tip: go easy in the first few miles.

# I LOVE THIS QUOTE

It is true that speed kills. In distance running, it kills anyone who does not have it.
—Brooks Johnson, famed U.S. track coach

I love this quote because as distance runners we sometimes abandon our speed. But the truth is, we still need it. If I had more speed at the end of the marathon in April 2009, I would be Boston Marathon Champion.

**KEEP EVERYTHING RELAXED, ESPECIALLY YOUR MIND:** Stay loose. Keep calm. Let the race come to you.

**BE PREPARED FOR PERIODS OF QUIET:** Sounds crazy to say this, but sometimes in a marathon you can feel almost . . . bored. But that's because a marathon is not a sprint. It's not a high-octane, bells-and-whistles extravaganza. You get some of that at the start and finish sometimes, and at points along the course (gotta love those bands!), but in most marathons—except for the New Yorks, the Bostons, the Londons— a lot of the course can be pretty quiet. Just you, the sound of your footfalls, and a few runners around you. Enjoy the peace and quiet. Embrace the time with your own thoughts.

237

**BRING A LIGHTWEIGHT CAMERA:** It's inevitable that in a marathon—especially if it's your first—you will see and feel things that you'll definitely want to document somehow, and a camera is your best bet. Wear a lightweight fannypack to carry it. I've heard of people taking self-portraits at every mile as a way to document their journey. That sounds pretty neat. Just be sure you're out of the way so that runners don't run you over.

**REMEMBER TO KEEP YOUR HEAD UP, WITH EYES LOOKING FORWARD:** And not just for the race photo. Too many marathoners get into that shuffle where they're looking down at their feet and would plow into a tree if it happened to be in the middle of the road. This isn't the most positive body language, for one thing. But more important, it's actually less efficient to run hunched over and looking down, as this will shorten your stride.

**RUN FOR YOUR MOM:** Marathons are pretty epic, but they're even more epic if you dedicate your race to a friend or family member. I think Mom deserves it. Or Dad.

## DEAR KARA

**I'm eighteen and I really want to do my first marathon, but when I told my parents about it, they were totally against it. They've never been runners and don't really get it. Should I do it anyway (I really want to!) or obey their wishes?**

A marathon is a big ask of your body, but you could be ready at eighteen. I would talk to your coach or your doctor and just make sure that they are in agreement that your body is ready. If they say that you will be fine, get them to speak with your parents. You want your parents to be involved and supportive of your running, not to push them further away.

**BUILD IN SOME WALKING BREAKS IF YOUR GOAL IS SIMPLY TO FINISH:** Used to be you were shunned, ridiculed, and tossed out of polite society altogether if you walked during a marathon. Not anymore. Now it's just considered smart racing strategy if your goal is to reach the finish line. The key is not to wait until you *have* to walk because you're tired. Take short walk breaks every mile or two starting from the beginning.

**STAY CALM AND EVEN-KEELED:** Of course, you will feel lots of emotions during a marathon. Like when you pass the wheelchair racer. Or when you lock eyes with the young man cheering for you. Or when you run right pass the lone bagpiper blasting "Scotland the Brave." And let's not even talk about the band cranking out a great rendition of Springsteen's "Born to Run." Savor all these moments. Store up the energy they give you. But just don't let them throw you off your pace. Steady. Steady. It's a long way to the finish.

**SEE THE OTHER COMPETITORS AS YOUR FRIENDS:** I mentioned this in the racing chapter, but it bears repeating. A marathon is a long race, so long in fact that your only real competitor is yourself. The idea is to beat the distance, not the person next to you. So hang in there, stay positive, and take positive energy from everyone around you.

**COUNT DOWN THE MILES STARTING AT MILE 20:** I have this tip in the racing chapter, but I wanted to include it again here, as it's such a great strategy for the latter, difficult stages of a marathon. Once you hit mile 20, say, "6 miles to go." At mile 21, say, "5 miles to go," and so on. Smaller numbers getting smaller is a much nicer thing for you to get your head around at this point in the race than larger numbers getting larger.

**BE STRONG WHEN THE COURSE TURNS AWAY FROM THE FINISH:** This is especially key near the end of the race. There are many marathon courses

239

## DEAR KARA

**My boyfriend was great about cheering me in my last marathon—he kept popping up everywhere on the course! But by the end, I was tired and annoyed and wanted him to just go away. Is this normal?**

This is totally normal! Although our loved ones want to support us and we totally appreciate it, there are times when it becomes too much and it begins to distract us and take away from our focus. Before your next race, talk to your boyfriend about only being at key parts in the race. Maybe the beginning, maybe a little boost in the middle, and maybe some cheering when things get tough around the 20-mile mark. Explain to him that you want his support, but that when you see him too much, it is distracting and takes you out of your "zone."

that have the unfortunate characteristic of turning away from the finish right when you thought you were getting close to the end. This can be tough psychologically, because your mind is telling you that you're going in the wrong direction, and what's going on? So simply be prepared for this, and be ready to combat it with a positive mantra, such as, "I'll soon turn for home," or, "Out and then back."

**TAKE IN FLUIDS *AND* CARBOHYDRATES:** In shorter races, water is all you need, and unless it's superhot, you probably don't even need that. But in half marathons and definitely in marathons, you need both fluid and energy replacement to keep your blood sugar up and your stored carbohydrates (glycogen) going to your hardworking muscles. Marathons provide sport drinks at the aid stations, which makes things easy for you, as they're premixed in the optimal ratio of water to carbohydrates (along with important electrolytes such as sodium and potassium). Figure to take in 5 to 8 ounces every 15 to 20 minutes of running.

**BELIEVE IN YOUR TRAINING:** Twenty-six plus miles is a long time to be running, and it's inevitable that doubts will creep in. Your main defense against these negative thoughts is to trust that you have trained properly. Again, having a positive mantra ready for when the going gets tough is a great idea. "I have trained, I am ready" is the type of strong, positive, brief message that works best.

## DEAR KARA

**I'm going to try to qualify for Boston next year. I need to run 3:40 or better. I think I'll be fine with the physical part of the training, but I'm a little worried if I'm tough enough for the race. Any specific things I can work on that will help?**

If you can train properly for a marathon, then you can run one. When you are doing your training runs for the marathon, make little mental notes about how much you are doing and how hard you are training. Keep these thoughts positive: "Look at me, finishing my long run, even though I am a little tired." On race day, keep going back to the training you did. You are certainly tough enough for the race!

**BUT ALSO REMEMBER THAT YOUR FAMILY WILL LOVE YOU NO MATTER WHAT:** This thought has been a great comfort to me in many races where I was racked with doubts, as I'm sure it has to countless runners. And it's true, so remember it if things get difficult.

**SHAKE OUT YOUR ARMS AND LEGS EVERY COUPLE OF MILES:** Running a marathon involves an incredible amount of repetitive motion, and your muscles and tendons can get in a "pace rut" if you don't wake them up from their stupor periodically. Just a quick flopping of the hands and arms should do it, along with a leg and foot shake.

**HOLD THE LINE IF THINGS GO BAD:** If you run enough marathons, eventually you'll run a real stinker. For whatever reason. Sometimes it has nothing to do with you, such as when the weather turns bad. But even at those times, you're the one who has to deal with it. If (when?) this happens to you, do damage control by inserting regular walk breaks. For example, if you totally hit the wall at mile 20, try not to pack it in and walk the rest of the way. You owe it to yourself and your months of training to try to tough it out if possible. So try walking for a minute, then running for a minute, then walking for a minute. Oftentimes, this sort of triage will help you recover enough to get moving again, and you will have limited the damage to your finish time.

**OR JUST RUN TO THE NEXT TREE:** This is another useful ploy to keep you going when fatigue hits hard. Break things up. Don't think about the 4 miles you still need to cover; just run to that fire truck parked a half mile up the road. Then run to the yellow house. Then to that cute guy standing alone on the curb. You can cover a lot of ground this way. Try it out.

**KEEP MOVING THROUGH THE FINISH-LINE AREA:** Fight the urge to stand around, chat, or even sit down right when you cross the finish line. Lots of runners will be coming in at big marathons, and traffic jams are fairly common. Sometimes it gets so bad that the crowd extends out in *front* of the finish line. Do your part and keep moving.

**REPLENISH THOSE CARBOHYDRATES, BUT GET SOME PROTEIN AS WELL:** The race will supply you with appropriate postrace food, so be sure to take advantage of it. Bagels, bananas, oranges, hot soup, yogurt—it's all good. Research has shown that four parts carbohydrates to one part protein is the optimal mix for reviving muscles and other soft tissues, and the sooner the better after finishing, even if you don't feel much like eating.

**WALK FOR A WHILE AFTER YOU FINISH:** Anecdotal evidence shows that you will recover faster from your marathon if you can do this. Get plenty of fluids also.

**REMEMBER TO GET YOUR THINGS AT THE BAG PICKUP AREA:** You'll be tired and maybe a little disoriented when you finish, so don't wander off to join your friends or family before getting your gear. Change into dry clothes if possible, or at least put on your sweats.

# I LOVE THIS QUOTE

I'm not going to run this again.

—Grete Waitz after winning her first of
nine New York City Marathons

I love this quote because this is how we all feel after finishing our first marathon. But seemingly overnight, we are planning the next one.

**LET THE PAMPERING BEGIN:** If you have the energy to hang out for the awards ceremony, try to do that. Otherwise, head home or to your hotel room and seriously chill for an hour or two after a rejuvenating shower. Put you feet up, maybe nap a while, and generally have your spouse of significant other wait on you hand and foot. Something to drink? Sure. Something to eat? Sure. Can I get you a blanket? Absolutely. And yes, a snooze may be just the thing.

**PLAN ON A CELEBRATORY MEAL AND A DRINK OR TWO ON RACE NIGHT:** Can you say 2,600 calories? That's how many extra you burned during the marathon, and that equates to a whole lot of Italian, Thai, Mexican, or Indian food—so go crazy. You deserve it. But be careful about the alcohol. The night after a marathon, after what you've put your body through, it doesn't take much to feel the effects. The term "cheap date" is definitely applicable here. Oh, and remember to wear your race medal to dinner!

**GET OUT THERE ANYWAY, EVEN IF YOU'RE DISAPPOINTED IN YOUR PERFORMANCE:** After a not-so-good marathon, it's natural to want to "crawl under a rock" in your bedroom or hotel room. Phooey. Give yourself a few hours to recover after the race, then hit the town. No matter how you finished—even if you *weren't* able to finish—you have a lot to celebrate.

**PLAN TO STAY OVERNIGHT AT THE HOTEL AFTER YOUR RACE AND/OR TAKE THE NEXT DAY OFF OF WORK OR SCHOOL:** Seriously, give yourself a little time to celebrate. Soak it in. Relax. You earned it. Plus, a flight or car ride home the night after a marathon can be tough on the legs ("Cramp! Ouch! Please! Stop the car!"). Give yourself a great night's sleep in a cozy hotel bed before heading home.

**CHECK YOUR RESULTS!** Thanks to electronic timing devices, many marathons are now able to post race results online the night of the race, so when you're back from dinner, check out your official time and how you placed. See how your club members did, or anyone from your area. And who knows—you may have qualified for the Boston Marathon, which is the only marathon in the world (outside of the Olympic Marathon and World Championships) that requires a qualifying time to enter. Check baa.org for the qualifying time you need.

**TAKE A FEW DAYS OFF TO BASK IN THE POSTRACE GLOW:** Hopefully this advice seems self-evident to you, but you'd be surprised by how many runners want to get out there the next day after a marathon for a run. Okay, maybe 1 or 2 easy miles if you absolutely have to, but otherwise figure on at least three or four days of total rest.

# DEAR KARA

**After my last marathon, I swear I was depressed for a month. How do you get through your postmarathon letdowns? Or do you not get them?**

I have gone through a period of depression after all of my marathons. I work so hard in preparation and it becomes my biggest focus for nearly three months. When it is all said and done, I'm sad that it is over. Each time I let myself be sad for a day or two and just accept that this particular journey has come to an end. Then I focus on enjoying my rest period and doing things that I am unable to do when I'm training hard. Finally, after my rest period is over (usually two weeks or so), I start planning my next race. Nothing gets you excited like a new race schedule and training plan.

**SHOW SOME RESPECT FOR DOMS:** Actually, delayed-onset muscle soreness will probably force you to pay heed. It happens to your muscles after an extended bout of repetitive exercise. And watch out: the soreness peaks at 24 to 48 hours after the bout of exercise, so a day or two after your marathon, you're going to be feeling it! Taking OTC painkillers like ibuprofen (Advil), acetaminophen (Tylenol), or naproxen sodium (Aleve) will help a little bit, but basically you have to just ride this out and it'll go away by itself. Meanwhile, best not to run with it. (It's not dangerous to do so, just painful.)

**DO A POSTMORT OF YOUR MARATHON EFFORT:** Within a week after your race, while things are still fresh, sit down with a pen and paper or on the computer and make some notes on what went right and what went wrong. Include your training period and the race itself. And be brutally honest. What would you do exactly the same next time? What would you change? Store your notes where you can find them once you start training for your next 26.2-miler.

**EXPECT TO FEEL THE LETDOWN:** Feeling down—sometimes *really* down—after a marathon is very common. After all, it was a big focus of your life for at least 2 to 3 months, and suddenly it's over. Now what? And it doesn't matter if it turned out well or not so well—the blues hit either way. Not to worry, since there are several things that can help:

- **Before your marathon, schedule a short, low-key, local race for about a month after the marathon.** This will give you something to look forward to.
- **Add a new cross-training exercise to your weekly exercise program.** Ever try Pilates? It's a fantastic complement to running. Learning something new will help distract you from your postmarathon malaise.
- **Make the most of your weekend mornings.** Chances are you spent many weekend mornings doing long runs leading up to your marathon. Sure, they gave you focus and they gave you purpose, but they were also a pain! Revel in being able to sleep in again. Read the Sunday paper. Start catching up on your reading. Go out for breakfast. Take a long bike ride with your husband or kids or training partner.

## DEAR KARA

**It blows me away that it took until 1984 for there to be a women's marathon in the Olympics. How dare they keep us from running that wonderful distance! What do you think about this?**

I was literally floored when I learned that there was no Olympic women's marathon until 1984. This was because of silly beliefs that have since been proven false. It was once believed that if a woman ran too hard, her uterus would fall out! For real! I'm so thankful that we have moved on from that and women of all ages can enjoy the benefits of running.

**DON'T RETURN TO RUNNING TOO SOON:** Just because the acute soreness from the race is gone, doesn't mean you're ready to jump back in to regular training. You may still feel flat (muscles take a while to recover), so take it easy for at least a couple of weeks. As mentioned in the racing chapter, a good rule of thumb is to do a really easy running day for every mile you raced, which translates to 26 days of easy running after a marathon.

**WHEN YOU DO RETURN, LEAVE THE WATCH (AND EXPECTATIONS) AT HOME:** Point being, just run free and easy for a while. No constraints, no strings attached. Don't even think of it as training. Just run. You earned it.

**ORDER THOSE RACE PHOTOS:** When the offer comes in the mail or via e-mail, say yes. But only if your eyes are open and you're not looking down at your watch. (And no, you *don't* look fat in your running outfit.)

# The World's Simplest Marathon Training Plan (15 Weeks)

Following is a nuts-and-bolts, highly effective training plan for a marathon. Before reading the plan, please review Chapter 7 to learn:

- The rationale behind training just three days a week
- How exactly to do your easy, hard, and long runs
- Where you need to be fitness-wise before starting this schedule
- How to convert the mileage listed in the plan to minutes of running, if that's your preference

|  | Tuesday | Thursday | Sunday |
|---|---|---|---|
| Week 1 | 4 miles (easy) | 2 X ½ miles (hard)* | 6 miles (long) |
| Week 2 | 4 | 2 X ½ | 7 |
| Week 3 | 4 | 2 X ½ | 8 |
| Week 4 | 4 | 3 X ½ | 9 |
| Week 5 | 4 | 3 X ½ | 10 |
| Week 6 | 4 | 3 X ½ | 12 |
| Week 7 | 4 | 4 X ½ | 14 |
| Week 8 | 5 | 4 X ½ | 12 |
| Week 9 | 5 | 4 X ½ | 16 |
| Week 10 | 5 | 5 X ½ | 12 |
| Week 11 | 5 | 5 X ½ | 18 |
| Week 12 | 5 | 5 X ½ | 12 |
| Week 13 | 5 | 6 X ½ | 20 |
| Week 14 | 5 | 6 X ½ | 12 |
| Week 15 | 5 | 3 X ½ | Marathon race |

* On each of your hard days, always start with 1 mile of very easy running, followed by the specified number of hard segments, always with ½ mile of very easy running between the hard segments. Always finish with 1 mile of easy cooldown. Thus, on your first hard day, you'll do: 1 mile easy, ½ mile hard, ½ mile easy, ½ mile hard, 1 mile cooldown.

# CHAPTER 9

# PREGNANCY AND NEW MOTHERHOOD

For much of my pregnancy, I felt conflicted emotionally and physically. Adam and I had always wanted children, but we were married nine years before Colt was born. My unusual career and some fertility issues meant bringing a child into the world wasn't easy for us. The recurring theme throughout my pregnancy? Tug of war. I felt like I was being pulled in two directions—by my running and my pregnancy.

At first it was really tough getting bigger and slower. I just kept thinking that I was a really tough person and should be able to push through everything. But in the end, I realized I was human. I was going to gain weight and I was going to slow down. In the first two trimesters, this was really difficult for me, but during the third trimester, I finally accepted the fact that it wasn't laziness—I was pregnant!

At the beginning of my first trimester, I was still doing short speed sessions but keeping my mileage way down. I wanted to make sure that the pregnancy took and that the embryo could fully attach to my uterus. Once we got past the ten-week mark, I started upping my mileage. I kept my speed workouts relatively short, but I let my mileage creep up. Halfway through the second trimester, I was up to 75 to 80 miles a week including two speed sessions. That turned out to be too much, as I ended up with a stress fracture in my lower back. I distinctly remember feeling like I needed to hit a certain mileage and running through the pain in my back, and a day later I couldn't even walk.

It was so silly—what did it matter if I ran 75 miles instead of 80? But I just couldn't shut off that competitive voice in my head. I do remember meeting Alberto to do 800s one day. The plan was to do them in 2:40, but I just kept going slower and slower until I was barely breaking 3 minutes. It was so frustrating. I cried afterward. I couldn't believe that I couldn't just push through, but that's the way it is—your body just won't let you do it. Again, it was so difficult for me to accept this.

I know that it seems contradictory to want a child so badly, then finally to get pregnant, yet to keep worrying so much about my running. But this is exactly how I was feeling. I've worked so hard to be the best runner I can be, and it was difficult feeling like I was letting all that slip. Being an elite runner is a 24-hour-a-day job. You are always doing something for your running, whether that's running, lifting weights, napping, getting a massage, eating right, seeing the chiropractor, and so on. As desperate as I was to be pregnant and have a child, I couldn't put aside those thoughts about becoming a better runner. It seems crazy now, but I wanted to be pregnant, and I wanted to be a perfect athlete, too. This was impossible to do, but I didn't have an answer.

Then that stress fracture happened, which enabled me to get a procedure done on my foot that I'd been needing for a while. These two things forced me to take a week off, which is when I finally started to relax a little bit and figure things out. I suddenly realized my body wasn't fat; it was just curved like the women in the baby books. My body had changed to hold on to the life inside of me. It's difficult to see the scale going up and up, but I finally realized it was what my body was created to do. Here I was, trying to remain as athletic as possible and not wanting to look pregnant. I finally realized how silly that was. For the rest of my pregnancy, I still had plenty of moments when I stressed about how slow I was running and how much weight I was gaining. But at the same time I had a deeper appreciation for my body and for the transformation that was taking place.

This is my promise to myself: If I am ever fortunate enough to get pregnant again, I will try to enjoy it more from the beginning. I feel like I really didn't fully appreciate the true beauty and the amazing time that it was until the eighth month. By that point, I was too big to do any serious workouts, so I ran for fun, for the pure joy of it. The rest of the day, I was a pregnant woman and I really loved it.

In the last couple of weeks before Colt was born, I didn't want it to end. I kept wishing that I could have another week or two. When I finally relaxed and appreciated the beauty of it all, I didn't want it to end.

As of this writing, Colt is just a month old. He is such a joy, and after nine years of marriage, he is truly a blessing for Adam and me. We have wanted a child for so long and we struggled to get pregnant, but now he is here and I get emotional just thinking about him.

However, I have to be honest and say that there is a part of me that is anxious. I feel overwhelmed at times when I think about "getting back to work" and all that I need to do. On the one hand, I feel like I need to be there for Colt all of the time. Yet I feel like I need to get back to my running career as well. The tug of war is back, the pull between the two passions of my life. I know that as Colt gets older and we get on more of a schedule, I will be able to manage more, but right now it's hard to juggle. I don't want to miss a thing with Colt, yet I miss training full-time and being a full-time dedicated athlete.

Thankfully, I'm also starting to realize that no one is perfect and that things will get a little messy at times. Yes, my training may suffer

251

a bit on occasion, but that is more than made up for by the happiness that Colt brings to my life. And if someone has to give Colt a bottle because my training ran late, he will survive and I'll be a better mother because I took the time to do something that makes me happy.

Yes, it's a tug of war all right. But I'm calmly determined that both sides are going to win.

# SMART, SENSIBLE TIPS TO HELP YOU RUN HEALTHY THROUGHOUT YOUR PREGNANCY AND AFTER THE BABY ARRIVES

A s you now know from my own story, running while you're pregnant isn't always easy. You may sometimes feel torn between that precious little wonder growing inside you, and that precious desire burning inside you to get your running body back! But hopefully you'll be better than I was about just letting the changes happen. And really, you don't have any choice. I was just being delusional in thinking I did.

But you aren't as thick-headed as me. A big part of the hang-up, of course, was that I make my living from running, and I felt as if my livelihood was being taken from me. Silly, I know, but true.

So my advice to you when your pregnancy comes is to calmly let your running take a backseat for a while. For however long it takes. Meanwhile, embrace your pregnancy for all it's worth.

Which isn't to say you need to stop running. Absolutely not, unless your doctor gives you a clear medical reason to do so. The following tips and strategies will help you continue to run happily, healthfully, and, ahem, *moderately*. Which in turn will help you and your baby in countless ways—both before and after delivery day.

**BE OKAY WITH THE WEIGHT GAIN:** Try not to obsess about the ever-higher number on the scale. I gained 35 pounds by the end of my pregnancy. But after Colt was born, it came off quickly. Nursing helped a lot, I am sure. It's the body's magic way of helping you lose the weight faster. But remember that weight serves a purpose while you're pregnant. Don't fear it, and try not to be frustrated by it. It is going toward the well-being of your child.

**CUSTOMIZE YOUR PREGNANCY AND POSTPARTUM EXERCISE PLANS:** Each woman experiences pregnancy in her own unique way. Follow general guidelines for exercise and nutrition, but make sure that these two key areas are also individualized for you by your health-care professional. As a runner, you will want to be sure your ob-gyn has some training in

## Four Common Myths

*Banish these worries once and for all, says my ob-gyn Robin Barrett, MD*

1. **Keep your pulse below 140.** *False.* Current guidelines based on the best medical studies give no heart-rate limits. Rather, use common sense, listen to your body, stay well hydrated, and never get overheated.
2. **You need to slow your pace.** *False.* However, it is common to feel more exertion when you run during pregnancy, because of the numerous cardiovascular changes your body is going through. You will probably slow down naturally as the pregnancy continues.
3. **No lifting your arms above your head during strength training.** *False.* It is fine to continue strength training. See Kara doing Pilates in the September 2010 *Runner's World* magazine!
4. **No lying on your back, and no abdominal work.** *False.* You can continue as long as you are comfortable, probably well into your second or even third trimester. If you are unable to lie on your back, you can continue to work your obliques on your side.

255

athletic medicine and can advise you *before* you start your pregnancy exercise program.

**GO WITH LARGER SIZES:** Early in your pregnancy, invest in some stretchy running clothes one size larger. This way, as your belly grows, it can stretch out the clothes. Also, invest in some good sports bras one size larger. Finally, consider going half a shoe size up as well, because your feet will probably swell (hey, everything does!). With all the swelling and the weight gain, you definitely want your feet to stay comfortable.

**TRY COMPRESSION TO EASE BREAST SORENESS:** If you have uncomfortable or painful breast tenderness when you run, try wrapping an ace bandage around your chest on top of the bra to increase the compression of the breasts so that they don't bounce as much.

**SUPPORT THE LOWER LEGS:** Speaking of swelling, compression socks were very helpful to me in the last few months of my pregnancy. I wore them every time I ran and I think they really helped me keep the swelling down in my legs.

**CONSIDER THE SURFACE YOU RUN ON:** When you're pregnant, you have looser ligaments, and thus may be more prone to overuse injuries and sprained ankles. So consider sticking to even surfaces like roads, sidewalks, or well-groomed trails. As pregnancy progresses, your body produces *relaxin* to get your pelvis ready to accomodate the growing fetus and delivery. These changes occasionally come with back or lower abdominal pain. An unlevel surface may exacerbate these musculoskeletal conditions, so hit a nice all-weather track if you really need an even surface.

**KEEP GOING ALL THE WAY THROUGH IF YOU CAN:** I ran 50 minutes the day I went into labor, which is proof that you can run your entire pregnancy. That said, I wasn't breaking any speed records during that 50 minutes—not even close! But I didn't care. It was just great to be out there doing what I love, and knowing it was helping me and my baby. The important thing to remember is that slowing down as you progress through your pregnancy is not only important but inevitable. You can't fight it and there's no reason to. Your body is changing dramatically and you don't want to end up injured.

## Why Run While You're Pregnant?

According to the American College of Obstetricians and Gynecologists (ACOG), continuing to run or do other aerobic activity during pregnancy for 30 minutes on most days of the week can:

- Reduce backaches, constipation, bloating, and swelling
- Prevent or treat gestational diabetes
- Increase your energy
- Improve your mood
- Improve your posture
- Improve muscle tone, strength, and endurance
- Help you sleep better
- Improve your ability to cope with labor pain

**MONITOR MORE CLOSELY:** If you do plan on running throughout your pregnancy, ask your doctor if you can have a few extra ultrasound measurements to make sure your baby is growing properly. This way you and your doctor can rest assured that you aren't doing anything that would cause stress to the baby.

**TRY TO STAY WITH THE EXERCISE—YOU'LL BE GLAD YOU DID:** The more that you can stick to an easy running and lifting routine toward the end of your pregnancy, the easier it will be to come back after you have the baby. Don't go crazy—just try to stick to a regular workout routine. You'll be amazed at how soon you are back running at your regular pace after the baby is born.

258

**STRENGTH TRAIN WITH CARE:** This may be a good time to emphasize toning of muscles rather than strength. Avoid strength exercises that strain the lower back muscles. During pregnancy, your back has increased loads and becomes more lordotic (swaybacked), which adds stress to the lower back muscles and ligaments. Avoid using heavy weights, particularly for the lower body, as these can increase your blood pressure and limit blood flow to the baby. Rather than doing leg presses, for example, do lunges and squats without weights.

**BE MINDFUL OF FLUID INTAKE:** While it's usually no big deal if you misjudge your water intake needs while running, getting dehydrated while

## IT WORKS FOR ME

**Pregnancy is tough on the bladder, which can make runs tricky.** I had a regular training run that went through the woods, so it was always easy to take a pit stop. Or you can do loops around your neighborhood so that you're never far from your house or apartment—or more to the point, your bathroom.

**If you are nursing and running, wear two sports bras!** Your breasts will be heavy and sore, so just double up. It doesn't look like you're wearing two bras, but the support makes all the difference in the world.

**If you're lucky enough to have a baby that falls asleep after nursing, take advantage of it!** Put on your running clothes, then nurse your baby. Then take off. Added benefits: Your breasts won't be full. You'll know for sure that your child won't be needing you for another feeding right away.

pregnant is a no-no. In early pregnancy, dehydration can cause over-heating, which can lead to organ development problems in the fetus. Later in pregnancy, dehydration can lead to preterm labor. So keep the liquids coming.

**BE GOOD TO YOUR PELVIC FLOOR MUSCLES:** Don't forget to do your Kegel exercises regularly during pregnancy and after delivery. You don't know where your pelvic floor muscles are exactly? You can identify them by using them to stop your "stream" when you pee. Once you know how it feels to use them, try for 15 repetitions 3 times per day. Do these in different positions, such as waiting for the light to change while you're driving, or while standing and waiting for an elevator, or while lying in bed. These muscles are working overtime carrying the weight of your developing fetus and may get overwhelmed when you run with a full bladder. Therefore, it's best to empty your bladder before you head out for a run.

**ALWAYS, *ALWAYS* LISTEN TO YOUR BODY:** Whether it's fatigue, or dizziness, or muscle weakness, or soreness in your back—pay attention! If you need a break from running, take it. Your body is already working hard to take care of the baby. There will be days when it just needs a break.

**PAY ATTENTION—AND REACT—TO SEVERE PAIN:** There are a few rare conditions in pregnant and postpartum women that deserve a medical checkup. For example, pregnant women may suffer a stress fracture in their pelvic bones, or even transient osteoporosis of the hip. So don't be too stoic if you are having severe pain. Get it checked out.

259

**KEEP THE PHONE HANDY:** In the last month of your pregnancy, always bring a cell phone or run with someone else who has one. You don't want to be out on the roads or on a trail without a phone and go into labor!

# Healthy Running: A Guide

*Robin Barrett, MD, was my ob-gyn during my pregnancy with Colt. An avid runner and marathoner herself, Portland, Oregon-based Dr. Barrett offers trimester-by-trimester tips for pregnant runners.*

### First Trimester

- Keep running. Running doesn't cause a miscarriage!
- Depending on your symptoms, your weekly mileage and pace may not change much this trimester.
- These common symptoms can interfere with running:

    **Fatigue:** Listen to your body. Cut down mileage or the number of days you run if you need to. You can increase both when you feel better.

    **Breast tenderness:** Wear two running bras or buy a larger size.

    **Nausea/vomiting:** Eat frequent snacks during the day. You can keep a protein bar by your bed for first thing in the morning. Try vitamin B6. You may need a prescription for antinausea medication from your ob-gyn.

    **Bleeding:** Stop running until evaluated by your provider. You may need to stop running until spotting stops, usually by 12 weeks.

### Second Trimester

- Keep running. Running doesn't cause preterm labor.
- By the end of the second trimester, you will probably need to decrease your weekly mileage and pace.
- These common symptoms can interfere with running:

**START BACK ONLY WHEN YOU ARE READY:** There is no prescribed time to get back to running after the birth of your child. There are so many variables, such as how tired you are, what your delivery was like, how much child care you have, and so on. Once you are out there, you will feel different. Labor and delivery have given you a wonderful "training

**Bladder pressure:** Empty your bladder before you leave the house. Pick routes with bathrooms or good ground cover!

**Pelvic pressure/discomfort:** You may need to alternate running with walking. You may need to start using more low-impact equipment—elliptical, bike—or swim more often.

**Contractions:** See the preceding tip for pelvic pressure. Call your provider if the contractions don't stop or you have any bleeding.

### Third Trimester

- Keep running. Running can help decrease the risk of gestational diabetes, preeclampsia (high blood pressure), macrosomia (large babies), long labor and delivery, and it can help speed recovery after your baby is born.
- Most women can continue to exercise in the third trimester. Many are still able to run, but weekly mileage and pace are very individualized at this point.
- These common symptoms can interfere with running:

    **Fatigue, contractions, bladder issues, pelvic pressure/discomfort:** See the tips in the second trimester section.

    **Joint pain/ligament instability:** You may need to wear support hose, pregnancy support underwear, abdominal supporters, and so on. You may also need to limit exercise to low impact.

    **Low amniotic fluid:** You may need to rest more and increase your fluid intake.

    **Low weight gain:** You can have the growth of the baby checked by ultrasound. You may need to rest more and drink more fluid.

261

event," but it will take several months for you to undo the marvelous cardiovascular feats you have performed, such as increasing your blood volume to accommodate the fetus. But just hang in there. Running is a wonderful way to combat the baby blues, to recover that prepregnancy weight, and to get back to setting goals for yourself.

**EASY DOES IT:** When returning to running after giving birth, be patient! Start with walking the first few days or weeks, and ease into running. Things have gotten stretched out and you need to let them tighten back up. And things need to heal as well. Staying on softer surfaces will help, but the main thing is to go easy.

**GET PLENTY OF CALCIUM:** The milk you are making to feed your baby uses some of the calcium in your bone reservoir, so be sure you are getting adequate calcium in your diet or supplement (aim for 1,000 mg a day). Oh, and research debunked the myth that babies don't like the breast milk of exercising moms, so don't let that keep you from getting out there for a run.

**DEAL WITH INCONTINENCE:** This is common after delivery and usually gets better during the first three months. A few things to try:

- Empty your bladder before running.
- Use a "super" pad while running.
- Do Kegel exercises. Abdominal strengthening exercises may also help.
- Consider pelvic physical therapy.
- Talk to your obstetric provider if the incontinence continues longer than three months. Don't be too embarrassed to do this!

**BE OKAY WITH SOME SEPARATION:** It's fine if you want to get away from your baby for a run. This will make you feel better, and you'll come back a better mother. Admittedly, I felt guilty doing this at first, so I would wait until Colt would fall asleep, then I'd run. That's fine, if that's what you need to do. But eventually it became okay to get out for a run even when he was awake.

**GET READY TO GET FASTER:** Some elite runners have cited a "motherhood effect," meaning they have improved their performance after having a baby. While this doesn't happen to everyone, many women believe the demands of pregnancy and childbirth make them stronger and heighten their pain threshold, which makes them able to train harder than they could before they got pregnant.

## Your Postpartum Plan

*When and how much you can run postpartum depends a lot on your delivery. Here's what to keep in mind, according to Dr. Barrett.*

**Easy Vaginal Delivery** (little or no perineal repair; minimal blood loss)
- Increase activity as you feel; there is no time frame or limits on when you can start running again.
- Check for bleeding or spotting with increased exercise. Stop running if you are bleeding more than one super pad per hour, and call your obstetric provider.
- Get enough fluids, especially if you are breastfeeding.

**Difficult Vaginal Delivery** (extensive perineal repair; increased blood loss)
- Let your body heal for at least two weeks.
- Start walking when you are up to it.
- Increase activity once pain and swelling are gone.
- Check for bleeding or spotting with increased exercise. Stop running if you are bleeding more than one large pad per hour, and call your obstetric provider.
- Get enough fluids, especially if you are breastfeeding.

**Cesarean Section Delivery**
- Let your body heal for at least two weeks.
- Start walking when you feel up to it.
- Be sure your incision is healing nicely before you start running again.
- Keep away from abdominal exercises for four weeks.
- Check for bleeding or spotting with increased exercise. Stop running if you are bleeding more than one large pad per hour, and call your obstetric provider.
- Get enough fluids, especially if you are breastfeeding.

263

# CHAPTER 10

# RUNNING FOR LIFE

I would not be the runner I am today if not for the generosity of other women runners like Lynn Jennings, Joan Samuelson, and Paula Radcliffe. I also would not be the runner I am today if not for the generosity of men like my grandpa, who got me started, and Coach Skogg, who nurtured my passion for running, and Adam, with whom I share that passion on the deepest level. But there is something special about the influence of one female on another. News flash: women are different from men, girls from boys! Females face a slightly different set of barriers and challenges as runners, and in life. Because we understand these barriers and challenges from the inside, women and girls are often better able to help other women and girls deal with them. When Joanie tells me that running doesn't have to take away from mothering, nor mothering from running, I feel deeply reassured, because she is a woman and she knows what she's talking about.

Women motivate and inspire one another uniquely, too. When Amy Yoder Begley pulls away from me in a workout, I dig deeper to stay with her than I dig to stay with my male training partners because Amy's a woman.

Recognizing all this, I try to have the same kind of influence on other females that Lynn, Joanie, Paula, and others have had on me. It comes naturally. In high school I wanted everyone on our team to enjoy their experience and stay involved. I hated it when any girl became discouraged and quit. My friend and fellow co-captain Amy Hill and I put a lot of effort into encouraging the other runners. We both felt instinctively that it was important to maintain a warm, friendly team environment where everyone felt included and welcomed. I remember how my friend Dharma used to get discouraged because she was always our seventh or eighth finisher in cross-country races, and only our top seven runners made varsity. I tried to pick her up by telling her that if she kept working hard, she could make the varsity cutoff, but I also reminded her that varsity wasn't everything. She could still enjoy training, racing, improving, and being part of the team even if she didn't make the cut.

At the University of Colorado my role was different. Everyone on the team was experienced, dedicated, and talented. No one needed a cheerleader. But the team did have leaders, and those leaders needed to set a good example. That's what I tried to do when I became a captain. I worked hard not only for my own sake but also because I wanted my teammates to see me working hard, whether healthy or injured.

The professional running world is even further removed from the high school running world on a psychological level. Even so, we're all human and we all suffer discouragement, self-doubt, and frustration sometimes. I've experienced my fair share of all of these feelings, and I know how helpful a word of encouragement or a gesture of support from one of my peers can be in dealing with low moments. I remember every small piece of support I've ever received from a runner I respect or admire. I can practically quote you the pep talks I've received from Carrie Tollefson, Amy Rudolph, Deena Kastor, and others.

In the past I couldn't imagine that a kind word from me could matter very much to another professional runner, but now I know it

265

can, so I never hold back when there's an opportunity. When I see a runner like my teammate Lauren Fleshman struggling with injuries, I tell her not to lose hope and to keep believing in her heart that she can come back better than ever, because it's true. I don't get hung up in remembering that Lauren has beaten me in the past and in worrying about a better-than-ever Lauren beating me again in the future. I want her to be successful, and I just think that helping her in any small way I can is the right thing to do, even if it does cost me at the finish line someday.

While I spend most of my time interacting with other professional runners, the people I most enjoy trying to help are new runners and young runners. They are just discovering a love for running, and running is such an overwhelmingly positive part of my life that I can't help but get a kick out of seeing the lives of others changed by it. I love going to events like the San Diego Rock 'n' Roll Marathon, where many of the participants are first-timers, and giving them whatever I can give to water the seed of their passion to run.

One thing I've observed, though, is that while I can inspire other runners, they don't need me to inspire them. They get the most inspiration from the friends and family members they run with every day. It doesn't take an Olympian to inspire other runners. You don't have to be fast or even experienced. That's why I encourage you to do all you can to water the seed of the love of running in those around you, even if you feel that the seed inside you has not yet fully sprouted.

I recognize that being an Olympian does create unique opportunities to have a positive influence. Running has given me a platform to inspire some people who are not runners and may never be. It has put my story in front of people and, for whatever reason, that story moves some who have no interest in running to reach out to me. I receive letters all the time from women, girls, men, and boys who don't run and do not seek running advice from me. One time I received a letter from a girl who lived in a town very close to my hometown of Duluth and who, like me, had lost her father. Those things, not running, were the basis of her connection to me. I wrote back and we've been corresponding ever since—and she still doesn't run!

I always write back. I'm a total sucker. It's beyond my power to not respond when a person in need reaches out to me. I have been so fortunate and blessed through running that I feel a responsibility to use my running to help others even when that help has nothing to do with running. It's often said that life is a marathon, and that's true enough, but it's also a relay. There is no finish line. Each generation passes the baton to the next. I try to live my life like a relay. It's not about me reaching some ultimate destination. It's about trying to always move in the right direction and sharing the secrets of my progress with others so that they can move forward, too, and share their secrets with yet more people, and so on. Inspiring others to run is my most obvious way of passing the relay baton, but not the only way.

In 2009 I went back to my junior high, the place where my passion to run was born, to speak to the student body. I was invited, of course, because I have become a successful runner, and I did talk about running, but my message was not that every child should run. My message was that every child should—and I believe every child can—find something he or she loves as much as I love running and make that thing a permanent part of his or her life.

Since becoming a mother, I have thought a lot about this stuff. My son has inherited the genes of two world-class runners and will be raised by two people who love running. So there's a pretty strong chance that he will become a runner, and he may even become a very good runner. Nothing would make Adam and me happier, but there are plenty of other things that would make us just as happy. We'll be just as happy if he falls in love with soccer or biology and uses his passion and gift to add something to the world.

Of course, who says a biologist can't run?

# FOOLPROOF STRATEGIES FOR KEEPING YOU FIT, LEAN, HAPPY, AND ENERGIZED FOR THE LONG RUN

said at the start of this book that I'm in love with running. It's been that way from the very beginning. And I expect it to be that way until the very end of my life.

Competition has been a huge part of my running since I started, but it will not be that way forever. I have some important goals I still want to accomplish—there's this little matter of the 2012 Olympic Marathon, for one—but eventually, competition won't be so important for me. When that happens, will I love running as much as ever? I believe so.

In fact, I've known for many years that my love for running was about way more than running races and being good at it. I just love how running makes me feel. Running is part of me and always will be. It makes me feel strong, beautiful, capable, humble, and grounded. It helps give me the courage and optimism to live a full and fulfilling life.

Which isn't to say I'm always ready to launch myself out the door on a run with a big smile on my face. Running isn't always fun, and it's not always easy. And I'm sure that in ten, twenty, or forty years from now, there will still be plenty of days when I feel like chucking it in and becoming a bowler. Or a couch potato. But in my heart of hearts, I know I'll be fine, thanks in part to some of the strategies you'll read about in this chapter.

Good luck and see you on the roads.

CUT YOURSELF A BREAK: If you're on the "Comeback Trail" after many years away from running, resist the urge to compare your present self to the college or high school standout you may have once been. That was then; this is now. And now is the time for reality-based running strategies that can still offer all sorts of satisfaction. For example, I know a recreational runner and mother of three who has had a great time setting a bunch of postmotherhood PRs at different distances and events. Come to think of it, she's just one child shy of having her own relay team!

# DEAR KARA

**I ran in college and loved it, then I stopped running. I just started back into it earlier this year after thirty years out of the sport, and I'm already getting a little bored with it. It's not the same! Help!**

Running for a college team is definitely different than going out and training on your own. In college you have races to train for and the friendships you have on the team. You might want to look at joining a local running club. You'll meet lots of new people, so you'll have that camaraderie you had back in college and you'll train together for events. It will give you that group/team/friendship feel of a college team.

PICK ONE AREA OF WEAKNESS EACH YEAR AND IMPROVE ON IT: This is actually a lot of fun and lends itself perfectly to a New Year's resolution every January. It also keeps things fresh, as you have a new focus every year. You're chronically tight and believe it contributes to your injuries? Dedicate yourself to getting more flexible, perhaps with a yoga class. Can't even do one push-up? Determine to strengthen your upper body with a calisthenic program, or buy a home dumbbell set. And so on.

**CONSIDER SUPPLEMENTS:** For years exercise experts have recommended taking glucosamine and chondroitin supplements to help ease any joint pain, especially in the knees, that may be associated with aging. Many runners swear by these supplements. They're not cheap, but they are available over the counter. The standard recommended daily dose is 1,500 milligrams for glucosamine and 1,200 milligrams for chrondroitin.

**RAMP UP YOUR CROSS-TRAINING:** Supplementing your running with other exercise is great for all sorts of reasons—recovering from injury, burning a few extra calories, keeping things varied, and so on—but it's especially good for master runners who may have lots of miles on their legs or who are a bit more injury prone. Regular, planned cross-training allows you to stay just as fit as you back off on the mileage a little bit. Don't get me wrong—I plan to run until the day I die, but I'm sure I'll continue with other exercise along the way.

# I LOVE THIS QUOTE

A woman naturally thinks about how she looks, and the marathon beats you up so much that you look terrible at the end. You do not happily go before the cameras. You just primp yourself as best you can and tell yourself, well, what can I do about it?
    —Uta Pippig, 1994 Boston and ING New York City Marathon winner

I love this quote because I also worry about how I look when I have to do press after a race. Racing takes a lot out of you and can leave you looking pretty bad. But, as Uta says, what can you do about it? The journey of the race was worth it!

**STRENGTH TRAIN TO HELP MAINTAIN MUSCLE AND BONE STRENGTH:** Running is excellent for the muscles and bones, but it helps to add strength work as well. Research has shown that bone density among women decreases at about 1 percent a year from age thirty onward (men aren't immune to this either, by the way). Strength training can slow this down significantly.

**MAINTAIN YOUR BALANCE:** Life balance is always important, of course, but in this case I'm talking about physical balance, which can become an issue for people in their fifties, sixties, and beyond. Regular running will help you a lot in this area, but activities such as yoga and tai chi are excellent as well and will bolster your mind and body in so many other ways. (Runners often overlook balance, but it's important to work on it at every age. After all, running is all about balance—you only have one foot on the ground at a time!)

**FREELY CHANGE GOALS:** Allow yourself to become a different type of runner as your life situation and experiences change. The running goals you had at twenty-five may not be suitable when you are forty-five or sixty-five. The key is to strive for goals that are in sync with your ability and environment at every stage of your life. Being overly nostalgic or stubborn doesn't work well when it comes to running goals!

**MIX IT UP:** Always look for new places to run, new people to run with, new races and race distances to try, and new training schemes with which to experiment. That's what makes running fun! Sure, some of those training schemes won't work too well, but some will. As the great runner–philosopher and essayist George Sheehan once wrote, every runner is an experiment of one. So go ahead and experiment.

**BE FLEXIBLE AND FORGIVING:** Reduce the pressure you put on yourself to get a run in every day. If every day works for you, fine. But there's no reason you have to do that. Days off are great for resting, allowing your body to recover, and reveling in the fact that you're a fit, healthy runner.

## DEAR KARA

**I'm a good runner now, but I'm still young. I'm worried that when I'm older and not very fast anymore, I'll lose my motivation for running. I don't think I'll be into this "just slow down and enjoy it" stuff. Any thoughts on this?**

I used to think that once I couldn't run fast, I would be ready to move on. But the more years that have gone by and that I've been blessed to do this sport, I realize that running is so much more than racing. Take it for what it is in your life and keep on your journey. If you get to the point where it isn't fulfilling, it is okay to move on! But don't worry about that now and let it take away from your enjoyment. Just take each day of running as it comes.

**BECOME A HEALTHY MOVING BODY:** If your exercise or fitness identity is too strictly focused on being a runner, setbacks such as injuries can be devastating. Consider developing a fitness identity that prioritizes regular daily physical activity, but not necessarily a specific mode of exercise. Running can still predominate in this framework, but it's great to have familiar options you can call on if need be.

**RUN FOR A DIFFERENT CAUSE EACH YEAR:** Most races have charities associated with them, or you can fund-raise for a charity on your own. When your running is also helping someone else, it can be a wonderful motivator.

**TUNE IN TO YOURSELF:** If you always run while listening to music, get in the habit of at least once a week turning off the music and listening to your breathing and foot strike. And I mean really listening to it, and nothing else. Focus on how your body feels and changes over the course of your run. Your senses can be more energizing and rhythmic than any song.

# I LOVE THIS QUOTE

I tell our runners to divide the race into thirds. Run the first part with your head, the middle part with your personality, and the last part with your heart.

—Mike Fanelli, club coach

I love this quote because it describes the perfect way to race, for any runner on any level.

**STRETCH TO MAINTAIN YOUR STRIDE:** Recent research on marathoners found that those in their sixties and beyond had significantly shorter running strides than younger marathoners. Stretching can help. Make it a regular part of your postrun routine, and emphasize the muscles and tendons in the front and back of the upper leg, as well as the lower back, which all affect your stride length.

**KEEP YOUR EXPECTATIONS HIGH:** There is no reason you should not be running into your eighties or nineties, as long as you are sensible about achieving a balanced lifestyle and the conditioning of your body. There is a multitude of research that states that cardiovascular exercise staves off a whole host of modern-day illnesses, and running is even used in the treatment of people with mental illnesses. Alter your goals to different competitions: try a triathlon or an ultrarace in a beautiful part of the world.

**REMEMBER TO MOVE!** Numerous studies have shown that because today's desk-top working and sedentary lifestyles are so far removed from the way we evolved, a myriad of long-term health-related issues can result.

We need to move a lot more. Running regularly is great, but it still doesn't take into account that our postural structure has to respond to gravity. If working at a computer, get in the habit of standing and stretching every hour. Try to stand as tall as possible and imagine space between each vertebra, and then move your spine in its four planes of movement: (1) flexion—roll down and touch your toes; (2) extension—feel like someone is pulling your head off your neck from behind; (3) rotation—keep your hips still and rotate your shoulders and neck as far as possible; (4) lateral flexion—do a side bend stretch.

**PAY ATTENTION TO POSTURE.** The design of perfect posture affords us the maximum chances of survival and performance. When the body is structurally free and balanced, the transfer from sensation to action is more efficient, and the spontaneous adjustments of the body are more harmonious. How do you want to perform—as the Leaning Tower of Pisa or the Empire State Building? Look at your own posture—can you achieve the natural plumb lines? Be aware of whether you are slouching, collapsed, whether your body is aligned, whether one shoulder is higher than the other or the pelvis is rotated too far. Start to stretch where you see your body may be tight or tense, and seek help from

275

bodywork professionals who are certified in Pilates, the Alexander technique, the Feldenkrais method, and so on.

**LEARN TO BREATHE EFFECTIVELY:** Shallow breathing can have horrendous effects on the immune system, especially when we are unaware of it. Joseph Pilates said that we should at least learn to breathe efficiently. The analogy he used was wringing a wet towel dry—squeeze every last drop of oxygen from your body by softening your rib cage and dropping your ribs toward your hips, and then fill your lungs by breathing into the sides and back of your rib cage. Practice daily, and notice how much easier your running becomes. If you can't manage this, seek professional help.

## DEAR KARA

**Do you ever feel too masculine when you're out running and sweating and all that?**

I don't ever feel too masculine, but I do embrace my feminine side. I like wearing pretty workout clothes and having gear that's "cute." I like the fact that I can push limits and athletic boundaries all while wearing a pink top and mascara.

**BE MINDFUL OF YOUR TECHNIQUE IN THE GYM:** Strength and conditioning routines that do not emphasize the correct starting positions are harmful because they reinforce the wrong postural position and therefore muscle length, making our muscles tighter in the long run. Ensure that you are in the correct neutral starting position and that you can maintain it with ease.

**STRETCH THE WHOLE BODY:** See stretching as a way to get the whole body back to its correct posture. Routines that involve parts of the body only, or holding stretches for a short period of time, are ineffective because we can't escape gravity. The pressure of gravity will keep returning us to our compressed, collapsed state, unless we correctly strengthen the body's foundations and lengthen where we are tight.

**DO PELVIC FLOOR EXERCISES:** These exercises are key for effective core stability and a stronger, more balanced body, but do not go overboard in doing exercises that are too hard. Gain an awareness of the pelvic floor and learn to maintain the contraction constantly, then combine it with effective breathing, and watch how easier life becomes.

**KEEP YOUR QUADS STRONG:** The large and powerful quadriceps muscle in the upper front of your leg is key for runners of all ages, as it helps propel you forward with every running step. But it's also key for knee health, as a strong, balanced quadriceps muscle helps keep the knee in its place and tracking properly. As you age and joints such as your knees get a tad more creaky, quad strength takes on much more importance.

**HIT THE POOL—BUT NOT FOR SWIMMING:** Pool running (sometimes called aqua jogging) may look a little funny, but it's effective. And if you think about it, it's almost the perfect exercise for master runners who want to run as much as ever yet keep their injury risk low. You're still running, so you get all those great aerobic benefits, but there's zero impact. If you're not a great swimmer and are hesitant about getting in the pool, buy a flotation belt. This will help with your buoyancy.

**RUN FOR HEALTH:** Running will boost your health at any age. Its positive effect on your health becomes even more profound as you age. It's incredible how many benefits it brings:

277

- Lowers heart disease risk
- Lowers risk of certain types of cancers

## DEAR KARA

**My hair and skin get dried out when I work out a lot and have to shower so much. What can I do?**

Sounds gross, but don't wash it as much. I don't wash my hair after my morning workout. I just rinse off in the shower; I don't always use soap. After my afternoon workout, I take a real shower. But avoiding washing my hair and soaping up after that first workout really prevents my skin and hair from drying out. If you work out once a day, try to skip a day of washing your hair twice a week. Just use a dry shampoo and wear it up!

- Reduces stress
- Improves sleep quality
- Boosts "good" HDL cholesterol levels and lowers "bad" LDL levels
- Lowers blood pressure

**RUN FOR WEIGHT CONTROL:** Controlling your weight gets a little tougher as you get older—sometimes a lot tougher! Running will help a lot. You burn about 100 calories a mile during running (no matter your speed). When you finish, you get the added benefit of a little caloric "afterburn" as well. Plus, most runners naturally tend to eat better, simply because it makes no sense to ruin the good work you've done out there on the run.

**RUN FOR YOUR KNEES:** If I had a dollar for every time I've heard that running is bad for your knees, I'd be a rich woman. I'm not sure when this myth got started, but it just won't go away, no matter how many times exercise physiologists and sports orthopedists refute it. But the fact is, running is good for your bones and joints—including your knees! Research has shown that among other things, regular movement such as running speeds the rate at which your body naturally replaces cartilage, which makes it stronger.

**RUN FOR YOUR BRAIN:** Countless studies have shown that regular aerobic-type exercise such as running can help keep your mind sharp as you age. Oh yes, I almost forgot: running boosts memory power as well.

**RUN FOR YOUR BONES:** Bone loss is more of a concern for women than men, especially after menopause. Running can help a lot. One study done a few years ago at the Melpomene Institute for Women's Research in Minnesota found that a group of active women between the ages of forty-six and eighty had a 25.6 percent higher bone density than a similarly aged group of women who were inactive. By the way, many women find that running improves their menopausal symptoms, including hot flashes and mood swings.

## DEAR KARA

**I used to hear that if you run for a lot of years, your breasts will sag. Is this true?**

This is not true. Your breasts will sag over time no matter what you do. Might as well be out there keeping the rest of your body fit!

**RUN FOR GREAT LIFELONG SEX:** Hey, good sex is all about blood flow, right? And there's nothing that gets your blood flowing more efficiently than running. Add to that the muscle tone that running provides, the confidence it gives you, and the physical attractiveness you gain from it, and it's no wonder runners make the best lovers. At any age!

**RUN FOR A LONGER LIFE:** That's right—studies have shown time and again that regular physical activity such as running can add years to your life. And not just years but *quality* years.

279

## DEAR KARA

**I've been running for a year now and it has really improved my self-image and my confidence. I love it. Unfortunately, my long-term boyfriend keeps putting me down about things, just like he always has. It's really getting on my nerves. What should I do?**

Break up with your boyfriend! He obviously doesn't appreciate you. Your running will help you through your breakup. You deserve better.

**GO BY FEEL:** Training schedules are important, and lots of runners depend on them to stay on track with their running. I certainly do. But once you've been in the running game for a while, there's a lot to say for just going with the flow each day. You feel good after the first 2 miles? Go a bit longer than you'd planned, or pick up the pace. You didn't get much sleep the night before and you've been dragging all day? Just do a couple miles. Tailoring your running in this way makes things go a lot more smoothly. You do what you can do each day. It's more . . . organic than following an abstract training schedule.

**TRY A TEAM RELAY RACE:** These are so much fun and there are lots of them around the country. The Hood to Coast relay (hoodtocoast .com) in Oregon and the Reach the Beach relay (rtbrelay.com) in New Hampshire are two of the largest and most successful, but there are many others. Basically it's you and eleven other people covering as much as 200 miles total, with each team member running three separate legs averaging about 7 miles each. Some teams are competitive; others are not—they're just trying to finish. Either way, it's a blast. Do it once and you'll be hooked.

**RUN FIRST THING IN THE MORNING ON YOUR BIRTHDAY EACH YEAR:** There is no better way to start your special day. It'll stay with you the rest of the day—I'm fit, I'm a runner, another great year to look forward to!

# I LOVE THIS QUOTE

They meant, of course, the first American *man*, so they should say so.
    —Doris Brown Heritage, on hearing Craig Virgin described as "the first American" to win a World Cross Country title. She had won five.

I love this quote because it shows how men are often seen as the real heroes in our sport. Meanwhile, we have women out there breaking barriers all of the time.

**GET YOUR KID (AND GRANDKID!) INTO RUNNING:** No need to do the hard sell. Just you getting out there most days of the week is setting such a great example, and chances are very good that your child will see how much running does for you—at which point the seed will be planted. Pick your spots in terms of when to ask him or her to come along. Wait for the teachable moment. Keep it low-key. It's your example that will have the most effect.

**BUY A NEW RUNNING OUTFIT EVERY TWO MONTHS:** Or maybe every three or four. The point being, this is a great way to give yourself a little motivation boost. You'll look better, which will make you feel better, which will make it way easier to get out the door.

**281**

**TREAT YOURSELF TO A PEDICURE AT LEAST EVERY THREE MONTHS:** Same deal as the new running clothes, except in this case you're thanking your feet for putting up with all that pounding. Running can be tough on

## DEAR KARA

**I have nice legs, but some women's running shorts seem so short. Do you think the longer or shorter style looks best on women? And what do you think about those new running skirts or "skorts"?**

I personally prefer a shorter pair of yoga-type shorts. They aren't tight enough to pinch anywhere, but I don't have any fabric getting in the way. I think that this type of short is flattering for most women, and you can get them in a length that you feel comfortable with. As for the controversial skort, I used to make fun of it. But then I wore one at a Nike photo shoot and loved it so much that I asked if I could keep it. It was really flattering! Now, I wouldn't be caught dead doing a hard track session or a race in it, but I was seen doing an easy jog around the Olympic Village in it and I got lots of compliments!

the feet and toes. Calluses. Blisters. Black toenails. General soreness. A pedicure is a nice way to pay your feet back for everything they do for you. Just be careful—sometimes you need some of the calluses you've built up during running. Be selective!

**THROW IN A MASSAGE AS WELL:** I get a massage every week. This is so important for keeping me injury-free and able to withstand the physical stress I put myself through during training. But massage is important for all runners. It helps keep your muscles and tendons healthy and supple, it'll definitely lower your injury risk, and it really feels good!

**RUN ACROSS THE UNITED STATES—OR AROUND THE WORLD:** A really fun way to stay motivated with your running is to literally map your progress each day. You can start by getting a map of your state, and after each of your runs, mark off on the map the distance you ran, slowly work-

## DEAR KARA

**It may seem silly, but I like to wear makeup when I run. I just want to look good. Is there a brand that you recommend, or a technique maybe, so that it doesn't run or look overdone?**

This isn't silly at all. Even though you are out there being an athlete, you still want to feel good about yourself, and sometimes that means looking good. I always wear a little mascara and lip gloss at the start of a race. It just makes me feel better. I know it's gone by the time I've run a marathon, but I feel good at the start.

One thing I have learned from running photo shoots is to use makeup that is oil and sweat-proof. You don't want makeup running down your face as you are running forward, and you don't want anything blocking your pores while you work up a sweat that might leave you with acne later.

ing your way down the highway (using a pen or marker) until you've crossed your state. Then move on to the next state, and eventually work your way to the Atlantic or Pacific—your choice. Have some fun with your journey. Take a day off when you reach the border of another state, for instance. Or prepare a food that your new state is famous for. And definitely celebrate when you finish your journey, perhaps by dedicating yourself to an even longer journey next time.

**DO A THANKSGIVING MORNING TURKEY TROT RACE:** These races are everywhere now and they're so fun and festive. Runners and spectators are excited about the day and meal to come, and the former are especially pleased because they have guilt-free eating to look forward to! I've heard a theory about why these races are so popular with runners, and I think it makes a lot of sense. The theory is twofold:

- **The shot across the bow.** Many runners see the Thanksgiving race as a way of laying down a marker, as if to say, "I will *not* let myself gain weight or become a sloth this holiday season, and this proves how serious I'm going to be about that." A line in the sand, if you will, beyond which weight gain will not cross.

- **The last hurrah.** For other runners, the Thursday morning turkey trot works in quite the opposite direction. That is, it marks the end of diligent, conscientious training for the year. One last artery-clearing blowout before settling blissfully into holiday repose until January 1, at which point you get back on the program. Until that time, you relax and give yourself permission to miss occasional workouts without guilt, and simply celebrate another year on the roads.

## DEAR KARA

**I don't like getting smelly when I run. Can you recommend a deodorant that works well for you?**

Everyone smells a little after they run. But I don't like to smell a lot, either. I use a strong deodorant before I go to bed, and during the day I use one that smells nice. The one I use at night gives me good wetness protection, and the one I use during the day keeps me smelling good. I personally use Dove Clinical Protection at night and Secret Invisible Solid Scent Expressions during the day.

**TAKE TWO WEEKS OFF COMPLETELY EACH YEAR:** Running is wonderful and I love it so much, but too much of anything isn't good. Sometimes you just need a complete break from it—a planned guilt-free break (much better than a forced break through injury!). I guarantee this will help you reenergize your mind and body and make you happier than ever to be a runner once you start back again. As for when to take your break? That's up to you. Wintertime works well for lots of runners. And by the way, you're not limited to just one two-week break a year. Do what works best for you.

**SAVE A DOLLAR FOR EVERY MILE YOU RUN:** Keep track of your mileage. At the end of each month, deposit your savings into a special running account that you use to contribute to your favorite charity. Or maybe it's your fund for buying running stuff. Or maybe you only use it for running-related travel. Or maybe it's a college savings fund for your child.

**BUY *CHARIOTS OF FIRE*:** It's still the best running movie ever made. You really need this movie in your home collection for those times when your motivation wanes. You'll get an instant jolt, I guarantee. By the way, there are some very cute guys in this movie as well, and their 1920s-era white running shorts and black leather running shoes are the best.

## DEAR KARA

**I've been looking for some good women's running blogs to help me stay inspired, but I haven't found any yet. Can you recommend some?** There are lots of blogs out there by women runners. On competitor.com you can read my thoughts and those of Deena Kastor and Marathon Mamma. Another great blog is by Sarah Bowmen Shea, the author of *Run Like a Mother.* Ask your friends what they are reading as well.

**TAKE JOY IN BEATING THE YOUNG FOLK:** I'm still young myself, but I'm looking forward to that time when I'm in my forties, fifties, and older when I'll be beating women (and men!) half my age in races. And that's not just me as an elite runner talking. If you stay fit and keep running and racing, you'll always beat plenty of young runners in races. For one thing, lots of races include walkers, so you know you'll finish ahead of them! Ahem, not that it's all about the competition or anything.

**SET A NEW SET OF PRS EVERY DECADE:** Runners love to keep track of their best times at different distances by knowing their PRs. But at a certain point, let's face it: it's not possible to keep setting PRs, because you slow down with age, no matter how hard you train. No problem. Just wipe the slate clean when you enter a new decade and start all over again. I actually know people who do this every year. A new year, a whole new set of PRs to go after. Works for me.

**BE MORE CONSCIENTIOUS ABOUT PAIN AND SORENESS:** The trusty adage to listen to your body is true at any age of running, but it becomes more important as you get older. You should listen and react if you feel pain or soreness that lingers more than a day. Back in high school and college, I could ignore pain and "run through it" without even taking a day off. But no way does that happen anymore. I pay close attention to anything that feels like it could develop into a full-blown injury. That means not running until the pain is gone, and getting some therapies started as well, such as extra stretching, massage, or a session or two with my active release technique (ART) person.

## DEAR KARA

**I've heard that sweating a lot can cause pimples and give you greasy hair. Is this true, and if so, what can I do about it?**

I'm no determatologist, but I find that when I am running a lot and am wearing a hat I do break out where the hat hits my forehead. What I have done that has worked great is to put a little acne cream on the areas that typically get irritated before I run. After I run, I immediately rinse my face off. This has really helped to keep my skin clear. As for the greasy hair, I have not found that to be true. I have long healthy hair and it takes daily beatings. I just make sure not to overwash it and to always let it fully dry.

**RUN AT NIGHT AT LEAST ONCE A MONTH:** Sure, wear reflective clothing, attach a blinking light to your shorts, and pick an extremely safe area, but then get out there. Go with a friend if you like. Running at night is a completely different sensation than daytime running. It's quiet. It's a little spooky sometimes. But maybe the best thing is, you feel like you're going much faster! When you're done, it's always a little more poignant returning to your cozy indoor abode—nighttime mission accomplished.

**STRETCH MORE:** You don't have to do anything elaborate. Even 5 minutes of light stretching after your runs can go a long way. Emphasize the legs, pelvic area, and lower back. And if you just can't get yourself to stretch per se, there's always yoga or Pilates, which are fabulous for improving flexibility and might be more fun for you.

## I LOVE THIS QUOTE

They're very tenacious. They're dedicated. Once a woman decides she's going to do something, she'll probably stick to it. The only problem with women is that if there's anything wrong with them, they won't tell you. They get out there and run on one leg. They don't moan and groan like a lot of men do.

—Arthur Lydiard, famed New Zealand running coach

I love this quote because this man truly understands women. We are determined and we will put up with a lot more pain than men!

**IGNORE THE NAYSAYERS:** Even now there are plenty of people out there who think runners are a little nuts. "Why do you do that?" they say. Or, "What's the point?" Or, "Aren't you getting a little old for that?" Or the classic, "Isn't that going to hurt your knees?" Just ignore these people. Or if you want to bother at all, tell them you love to run, you will always run, you get a huge amount out of it, and they would, too, if they gave it a chance.

**RUN WITH YOUNG PEOPLE:** It can be fun and exciting to run with much younger runners than yourself. You'll glean insights you wouldn't normally get from your peers, and it helps keep you young as well.

**REVISIT THAT MARATHON THING PERIODICALLY:** Marathons are fantastic in so many ways, but after a while they do take a toll. Sometimes it's just the training that gets tougher to fit in and get motivated for, even if the race itself retains all the magic it ever held for you. But you don't have to keep running marathons until you drop! Instead, consider this: How about making the half marathon your "new" marathon? It takes half the time to train for, race day doesn't take nearly as much out of you, and you recover twice as fast. So there you go—half the distance, twice the fun.

## DEAR KARA

**Do you think it's fair that elite women runners are sometimes gender tested but male elites aren't?**
Well, that is tricky, because it wouldn't be much of a benefit for a woman to compete as a man, whereas a man competing as a woman gets an unfair advantage. I think it's a part of life. Just like the way I don't love getting drug tested all of the time, but that is what it takes to keep the sport clean, so I fully support the drug testing policies. Sadly, there are men who try to compete as women, and unless you test for it, you could never catch it.

**DO NOT GO GENTLE INTO THAT GOOD NIGHT:** To take inspiration from the Welsh writer Dylan Thomas, maybe race competition is your thing, and maybe it will always be your thing. That's fine! There's no one saying you need to hang up your racing spikes at thirty, or forty, or sixty. (Even if they are saying it, just ignore them.) If you love to race and plan to keep doing do it your whole life, you might be interested in age-graded races or an age-graded calculator. Age grading makes use of a formula that puts everyone on a level playing field regardless of gender or age. So, for example, using an age-grading calculator, a sixty-five-year-old woman running 40 minutes for a 5K is actually "faster" than a twenty-five-year-old woman running 29 minutes for a 5K. That's good racing incentive as you get older.

**INCORPORATE MORE HILLS IF YOU'RE TIRED OF REGULAR SPEEDWORK:** Over the years you may get sick of more standard speedy stuff such as intervals, *fartlek,* or tempo. No problem—just do hills instead. Hills get your heartbeat up high, but with less wear and tear than doing speedwork on the track. U.S. Olympic Marathon great Frank Shorter once called hills "speedwork in disguise." He was right.

# COACH SALAZAR ON GOING WITH THE FLOW

*Alberto Salazar has been my head coach at the Nike Oregon Project in Portland, Oregon, since 2004. During the early 1980s he was one of the best distance runners in the world—probably the best. In the remarkable year of 1982, when he was just twenty-four, Salazar won the Boston and New York City marathons and set American track records in the 5,000 and 10,000 meters. Does he miss those speedy days? Not a bit. His thoughts on running and aging:*

289

**BE WILLING TO CHANGE PRIORITIES:** I run 3 to 4 miles a day now and love it. I do it for health, stress relief, and fun. There is no pressure to run at a certain time of the day and no pressure to go fast.

**JUST KEEP IT MOVING:** I average about 8:30 to 9 minutes per mile, but I rarely keep track of my time. It's really just about getting out there and moving for half an hour.

**BE REASONABLE:** Since my heart attack in 2007, my doctor says he'd rather I run slow than fast. So I run slow. He says about 110 beats a minute during running is right for me, given that my resting heart rate is 50. So I don't go any higher than 110. I'm very pragmatic about it.

**RUN IN GOOD TIMES AND BAD:** Running does so much for me that I sometimes do it even when I'm sick. I just go slower. Never more than 4 miles, though.

**BEWARE WHAT YOU SIGN ON FOR:** I don't run hard anymore. Why should I? The last time I did, it was for a 10-mile race in Minnesota a few years ago. Kara was running it also. I wanted to run under 70 minutes, which is 7-minute miles. So I did the training for it—intervals, *fartlek*, the whole bit—and I hated it. I broke 70 in the race, but I have absolutely no desire to train or race like that again.

**DON'T LOOK BACK:** Sometimes people say to me that they really miss their younger years when they were faster. I don't get that. I tell them just run slower and be fine with that. I tell them I used to run sub-5-minute miles for an entire marathon. I held the marathon world record. Now I'm slow—and I'm fine with that!

# I LOVE THIS QUOTE

Once you leave this tunnel, your life will be changed forever.
　　　　—Joan Benoit's thoughts prior to entering the Olympic stadium in
　　L.A. en route to winning the first-ever Olympic Marathon for women

I love this quote. It gives me chills. Joanie was so aware of what her accomplishment was going to do for women. And she wasn't afraid; she met it head on.

# PHOTO CREDITS

Photographs on pages 3, 41, 77, and 207 courtesy of Patty Wheeler.

Photograph on page 140 courtesy of Kara Goucher.

Photographs on pages 16, 22, 31, 101, 109, and 229 by Guy Helson.

Photographs on pages 60, 80, 118, 127, 196, and 221 courtesy of
   PhotoRun.

Photographs on pages 192 and 224 courtesy of New York Road Runners.

# INDEX

297

301

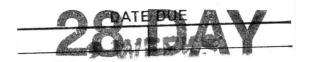